This is a rich and informative book that everyone who has an interest in maternal mental health should read.

— *Dr Gwen Adshead, Psychiatrist and Psychotherapist*

A clinically rigorous book about perinatal OCD, written with palpable warmth. Timely recognition and empathetic care can transform lives; this book offers both.

— *Dr Sabina Dosani MBBS MSc PhD FRCPsych, Consultant Child and Adolescent Psychiatrist*

Dr Chrissy Jayarajah has set out to tackle gaps in understanding, and this easy-to-read book should be read by all who work with mothers and babies.

— *Professor Lynne M Drummond, Honorary Consultant, SW London and St George's NHS Trust and Visiting Professor, University of Hertfordshire*

Training gold – crisp, stigma-shattering and deeply practical – this book helps clinicians spot perinatal OCD 'hidden in broad daylight'.

— *Margherita Zenoni, Women in Neuroscience UK Rising Star of the Year 2025, PhD Candidate at University of Cambridge, Head of Fundraising at Orchard OCD*

Understanding Perinatal OCD

of related interest

Can I tell you about OCD?
A Guide for Friends, Family and Professionals
Amita Jassi
Illustrated by Sarah Hull
Foreword by Isobel Heyman
ISBN 978 1 84905 381 5
eISBN 978 0 85700 736 0

Supporting Parents and Families with Perinatal Mental Health and Wellbeing
An Introduction for Professionals
Dr Jane Hanley and Mark Williams
ISBN 978 1 83997 037 5
eISBN 978 1 83997 038 2

Understanding OCD
A Guide for Parents and Professionals
Edited by Adam B. Lewin and Eric A. Storch
ISBN 978 1 84905 783 7
eISBN 978 1 78450 026 9

UNDERSTANDING PERINATAL OCD

A Guide for Professionals

Dr Chrissy Jayarajah

Jessica Kingsley Publishers
London and Philadelphia

First published in Great Britain in 2026 by Jessica Kingsley Publishers
An imprint of John Murray Publishing Group

2

A CIP catalogue record for this title is available from the British Library and the Library of Congress

ISBN 978 1 83997 209 6
eISBN 978 1 83997 210 2

Printed and bound in the United States by Integrated Books International

Jessica Kingsley Publishers' policy is to use papers that are natural, renewable and recyclable products and made from wood grown in sustainable forests. The logging and manufacturing processes are expected to conform to the environmental regulations of the country of origin.

Jessica Kingsley Publishers
Carmelite House
50 Victoria Embankment
London EC4Y 0DZ

www.jkp.com

John Murray Publishing Group
Part of Hodder & Stoughton Ltd
An Hachette Company

The authorised representative in the EEA is Hachette Ireland,
8 Castlecourt Centre, Dublin 15, D15 XTP3, Ireland (email: info@hbgi.ie)

I dedicate this book and all that I am to my two daughters, Ruby Maya and Ivy Gaia, who have taught me what is to be a mother;

to my husband Wyman, for showing me what it means to love and be loved;

and

to my parents, who first showed me the meaning of love and laid the foundation for everything I am.

In loving memory of Mummy,

'For you created my inmost being; you knit me together in my mother's womb.'

(Psalm 139 v13)

Contents

A note on terminology – The terms 'sex' and 'gender' are used interchangeably in this book to reflect the inconsistencies noted in the limited evidence-based literature on this topic over the past 20 years. In this context, 'sex' refers to the biological determinants, while 'gender' relates to the social definitions assigned at birth. I acknowledge the recent broader cultural and politically relevant discussions surrounding gender, particularly the modern understanding of gender fluidity and non-binary identification (Pryzgoda & Chrisler 2000). Similarly, the term 'mother' is predominantly used in the text to mirror the focus of much of the existing literature, but it applies to all birthing people and/or primary caregivers during this vulnerable period.

In the same vein, I wish to begin by reflecting on the term 'perinatal'. Although most commonly associated with women and mothers, it can be used in various contexts and to describe different individuals providing care during a child's early years. This includes, but is not limited to, fathers, grandparents, older siblings, and non-biological carers such as adoptive parents, foster carers, and those within blended families. I also extend the definition to include birthing people such as transgender mothers. More research is needed to better understand perinatal OCD, especially in those who bear parental responsibilities, as they navigate the subtle but significant differences in a society that, for the most part, maintains a somewhat outdated 'two-dimensional' understanding of what 'mother' and 'family' truly mean.

Finally, I generally use the traditional reference term 'patient' for the individual receiving medical care; however, I acknowledge that in clinical practice other descriptive terms exist, including 'service user' and 'client', and that these terms may be adopted depending on individual preference and local practices.

Prologue

My first encounter with obsessive-compulsive disorder (OCD) was on my very first night shift as a junior doctor in Accident and Emergency (A&E). Although I was working in medicine at the time, everyone knew I was an aspiring psychiatrist, so I was naturally assigned all the mental health reviews on call. While some might feel uneasy, I secretly enjoyed this apparent bias. I found meeting with these patients a far more interesting way to spend a night shift than clerking numerous people in triage with suspected chest infections or headaches.

I'm unsure why Alice (not her real name) had come to the emergency department, but the story was that she was worried she might stab her five-year-old son. At first glance, the casualty records confused a young and inexperienced medic like me. Alice told me she was having intrusive thoughts of accidentally stabbing her son with a knife while making dinner or pushing him into traffic during the school run. She also experienced visual flashing images of her son covered in blood. I diligently wrote the history verbatim in my notes as my heart skipped a beat while I tried to mentally catch up with what she was telling me. I had no idea what to do or say to console her tears.

Given my concerns about the child (who was being cared for by his father at home at the time of the assessment), I thought it would be sensible (on the advice of the medical registrar, who was equally confused) to contact the on-call social worker. However, we couldn't get through in the early morning hours. He then suggested bleeping the senior psychiatrist on call as this was 'clearly psych'. Fortunately, the psychiatrist immediately recognised that it was a clear presentation of OCD and provided some sensible advice. We devised a safe care plan together, which allowed Alice to leave the emergency department with support in place and to be followed up in the community by the mental health team, where she could receive adequate and appropriate treatment.

I have often wondered about Alice. At the time, I certainly had no idea this could be obsessive-compulsive disorder. Now, with the advantage of experience and hindsight, I believe that this woman would have been living with the condition for a long time – possibly since her pregnancy – and that her symptoms escalated during the postnatal period and remained untreated until she reached breaking point years later, bringing herself to A&E.

Sadly, Alice's story is all too common. Perinatal OCD is rarely talked about, let alone identified. When it is recognised, it is often wrongly diagnosed as postnatal depression or anxiety. Patients are led down a path that never truly tackles the underlying cause. Also, as in this patient's case, inexperienced practitioners (like I once was) may react without fully understanding the nature of the condition. This is because the patient has no real intention of harming others and does not pose a risk to others despite the intrusive thoughts or disturbing visual images. There is also the unspoken truth that the stigma around mental health remains a problem. The stigma exists not just in social settings and communities but also within healthcare services and, dare I say, among some staff members.

During my core psychiatric training, I was fortunate enough to be assigned to the National OCD/BDD Unit in Tooting, South London. I recall someone suggesting the role to me as a valuable learning opportunity, as it involved being part of a service that operated at both national and local levels within the NHS. What I didn't expect was the experience of working with patients with the most severe obsessive-compulsive disorder I had ever seen.

I later learned that the World Health Organization categorises OCD as one of the top five disabling conditions affecting women of childbearing age. I am fortunate to have been guided by some of the best psychiatrists in the UK, who have dedicated their careers to improving the lives of those with OCD – namely Dr Lynne Drummond and Dr Himanshu Tyagi. They are not only colleagues but also lifelong mentors who exemplify excellence as clinical academics. Although I ventured into perinatal psychiatry, my time on the OCD Unit and the connections I formed there have stayed with me throughout my career. I began to gravitate towards places and activities that intertwined obsessive-compulsive disorder and perinatal mental health. This is something I did not fully see during my training.

I was delighted to learn about the wonderful UK-based charity Maternal OCD. Near the end of my training, around the time I started exploring 'med Twitter', I had the opportunity to join them in hosting a cosy Twitter 'chat' evening focused on perinatal OCD. While we could have easily held this event from the comfort of our own homes, we chose to gather on a dark and rainy October evening during National OCD Week. To this day, sitting around a small table and engaging with questions in the chat remains one of my most cherished memories. It truly made me realise that this was more than just a 'job' – it was a calling. Later on, I was honoured to be invited to serve as a voluntary scientific adviser for the charity, where I could contribute my knowledge on medication use during pregnancy and breastfeeding to support individuals with perinatal OCD.

The blurry boundaries between professional and personal life do not faze me, as I am very much living and experiencing the 'perinatal period' myself. I wrote this book during a time in my life when I became a new mother once again to my youngest daughter and joined the 'two under two' club. The book proposal was sent and accepted just before I went into labour! I thought nothing of it at the time, but in hindsight it has been the most wonderful labour of love. I fully engaged with maternity leave, watched my young preschool children grow, and eventually returned to work in the NHS full-time. Somehow, I also managed to find stolen moments between naps and early morning feeds to write much of this work. It was an opportunity to exercise my mind and, for a moment, to escape from the huge demands of motherhood and clinical responsibilities.

My reason for writing this book is my unwavering belief that understanding perinatal OCD is everyone's responsibility. My aim is to educate and empower all frontline staff who may encounter a mother and her child, including but not limited to midwives, obstetricians, junior doctors, neonatal nurses, lactation specialists, pharmacists, mental health nurses, health visitors, undergraduate students, physiotherapists, occupational therapists, GPs, social workers, A&E doctors, nursery workers, psychologists... the list continues. Those working directly with women during pregnancy and the postnatal period are likely to meet them at various stages of this journey. During this time – 1001 days (from conception to the child's second birthday) – a woman will have more contact with health professionals than at any other stage in her life, providing opportunities to identify and refer concerns if needed. The perinatal period offers a real chance for clinicians to make a positive impact. I hope that, by reading this book and learning about this common yet overlooked condition, you will be able to recognise the signs and symptoms of perinatal OCD, improve your therapeutic skills in helping women share their fears, and gain confidence in signposting to suitable services.

As I often mention during my teaching seminars, no one expects you to become a specialist overnight. However, having a basic understanding of what to look for is essential when encountering these vulnerable women. It can mean the difference between someone suffering silently for years and someone receiving prompt treatment. This condition can be fully and quickly treated with simple measures, such as medication and psychological therapy.

Although this book is primarily aimed at clinicians, I also encourage those affected by perinatal OCD and their families to read it. It aims to enhance their understanding of this distinctive condition and give them the knowledge and confidence to manage their own mental health needs.

In Part 1, I begin the book with an acknowledgement that the responsibilities of parenting are a breeding ground for worry; where intrusive thoughts and being overcautious (particularly for first-time parents) is not unusual. I argue that OCD presenting in the perinatal period is a unique condition with distinguishing features impacting on the mother and infant. Sadly, symptoms are often minimised or mistaken, and the condition remains under-reported, under-detected, and under-diagnosed.

In Part 2, I focus our attention on motherhood, mental health and OCD. We dive deep into unravelling the concept of maternal love and evolution of matrescence – the biological, hormonal, psychological, and social shift in becoming a mother. This is coupled with a socio-political commentary on how mothers have been treated over the decades and the impossible standards placed upon them. I also explore the narrative around being the 'perfect' mother, and the fine line between perfectionism, OCD and mental health in motherhood.

In Part 3, we further our understanding of perinatal OCD: the neurobiological basis of the illness and the historical aspects of OCD and perinatal mental illness, along with how it has shaped our view of the condition in the modern practice. I explore how OCD can affect different groups in specific situations (such as in fathers, those in same-sex relationships or of ethnic minority groups). I also explore the interface of perinatal OCD with religious and spiritual beliefs, and aspects of mental health law, including mental capacity and safeguarding.

In Part 4, I focus on classification and assessment of perinatal OCD to ensure an accurate diagnosis, and on the personal and systemic barriers that may hinder this. An inaccurate diagnosis can lead to a cascade of mismanagement and distress with potentially serious consequences for the patient and their family. I explore several differential diagnoses that OCD can often be mislabelled as in clinical practice, such as postnatal depression, health anxiety, psychosis, or body dysmorphia. Although, in reality, patients may present with dual diagnoses (such as autism spectrum disorder and OCD), this outline can be helpful in tailoring the specific needs of the patient to ensure that the appropriate treatment pathway is followed.

Part 5 is devoted to the treatment of perinatal OCD. Here, we'll look at aspects of treatment modality (talking therapies, medication, and newer techniques) and how aspects of treatment may be governed by the severity of illness and treatment location (community or inpatient support). I include detailed information on questions that come up consistently in clinical practice, such as the safety concerns of medication use in pregnancy and breastfeeding, but I have made a conscious effort to avoid medical jargon where possible.

Throughout this book, I share examples of perinatal OCD along with stories from my clinical practice to illustrate key themes discussed. I keep these case vignettes somewhat vague because the specific details are less important. Any identifiable details have been fictionalised to protect individuals' privacy. What matters most are these personal stories, which emphasise the importance of stepping back to consider the broader context of a person's life and understanding that their symptoms extend beyond mere diagnostic checklists.

PART 1

INTRODUCTION TO PERINATAL OCD, ITS SYMPTOMATOLOGY, AND SUBTHEMES

In Part 1, we will examine the fundamentals of perinatal OCD. I explore the spectrum of worries and intrusive thoughts that are common among new parents, and how to distinguish these natural and expected concerns from a diagnosis of perinatal OCD. I summarise some of the latest research supporting the argument that perinatal OCD has unique features, distinguishing it from generalised OCD or from other perinatal mental health issues. In Chapter 3, we delve into various themes of perinatal OCD such as FEAR OF HARM/AGGRESSION, FEAR OF CONTAMINATION, and SEXUAL/RELATIONSHIP OCD. I hypothesise that these themes are not mutually exclusive but rather interwoven during the perinatal period, which makes identification and management more challenging in clinical practice.

CHAPTER 1

Defining Perinatal OCD

WHAT IS OCD?

Obsessive-compulsive disorder (OCD) is a mental health condition. It is defined by symptoms of obsessions and compulsions that are severe enough to affect one's daily life and relationships.

- *Obsessions* are unwanted intrusive (and sometimes disturbing) thoughts, urges, or images that trigger negative feelings and distress.
- *Compulsions* are the behaviours, routines, and rituals one will engage in to reduce or neutralise distress that the obsessions have caused.

One of the challenges of OCD is its cyclical nature. Compulsions often only offer temporary relief, forcing individuals to repeat compulsive behaviours to keep counteracting the obsessions. The term 'obsession' comes from the Latin *obsidere*, meaning 'to besiege' (OCD-UK 2025b) This provides a quite unusual yet intriguing way to visualise obsessional beliefs, since the strict definition of 'besiege' is to surround a place with armed forces to capture it or force surrender. Conversely, 'compulsion', meaning 'a drive or urge', derives from the Latin verb *compellere* (*com* – 'with', 'together', and *pellere* – 'to drive'). These terms help us to understand the true gravity of this debilitating condition. Around 1 to 3% of the general population is thought to experience OCD at some point in their lives (Mathes, Morabito, & Schmidt 2019). OCD can be categorised into different subthemes, including individuals who experience both obsessive and compulsive symptoms, as well as those who experience only obsessional symptoms (often called 'pure O'), which will be discussed in Chapter 3 (Zambaldi et al. 2009).

WHAT IS PERINATAL OCD?

Perinatal OCD is simply OCD occurring during the perinatal period, from conception up until 12 months postnatal.[1] The term 'perinatal' is inclusive of OCD in pregnancy (antenatal) and postnatal OCD, though in practice several different terms, including perinatal, antenatal, maternal, postpartum, and postnatal OCD, may be used interchangeably. In clinical settings, as with all perinatal mental health conditions, patients can be categorised into:

- those who have pre-existing OCD
- those who experience symptoms for the first time during pregnancy or following delivery, who are referred to as having 'new-onset' perinatal OCD.

The symptoms of OCD remain similar, but in perinatal OCD (both pre-existing and new onset), there is often a dominance of obsessive fixation on the care needs of the baby, worsened by the additional responsibilities of being a parent to an infant.

The incidence and prevalence of OCD are now understood to be much higher than previously believed. A recent Canadian study revealed that cases of perinatal OCD are significantly more common than earlier estimates. In pregnancy, 7.8% of pregnant women exhibited symptoms consistent with an OCD diagnosis, and this doubled when including those in the postnatal period (Fairbrother et al. 2021). The study also identified 49 new cases of OCD within six months after birth out of 535 women, equating to a total cumulative incidence of 9% for the condition. However, even these elevated figures are probably an underestimate, as the questionnaires used in the study are general adult OCD screening tools not specifically tailored for perinatal OCD. Therefore, it is vital that clinicians working with women during the perinatal period have a thorough

1 Some NHS perinatal mental health services have extended the definition of the perinatal period to two years postnatal.

understanding of how mental health issues, particularly perinatal OCD, present in this context to prevent misdiagnosis or mistreatment, or completely missing the condition.

Despite the rising occurrence of OCD presentations during the perinatal period, including new cases, it has received relatively little attention in both academic research and clinical practice compared to postnatal depression, which is widely recognised and understood in comparison (House et al. 2016). In fact, 'postpartum depression' is often used as a general term for emotional and psychological issues during the perinatal period. It is also true that these conditions can occur together. Chaudron and Nirodi (2010) note that the presence of obsessive-compulsive symptoms and OCD can affect subsequent postnatal depression. In Chapter 3, we will examine the main themes that emerge in those experiencing perinatal OCD, with differential diagnoses discussed in Part 4. However, before exploring different conditions, we need first to understand the continuum of natural fears, intrusive thoughts, and obsessive-compulsive symptoms that are common in the perinatal period.

INTRUSIVE THOUGHTS

On average, humans have 6000 thoughts a day, with a tendency towards negative thoughts (although this can be overridden if recognised). To receive an OCD diagnosis, one must experience unwanted intrusive thoughts. However, not all unwanted intrusive thoughts indicate OCD. These thoughts are not only common but become more frequent after having a baby. Abramowitz, Schwartz, and Moore (2003a) surveyed the inner thoughts of 600 healthy mothers and fathers within a year of having their first child. They categorised seven themes of intrusive thoughts, including thoughts of suffocation or sudden infant death syndrome (SIDS), accidents, unintentional harm or urges, losing the infant (such as someone stealing the baby), serious illness, contamination, and unacceptable sexual thoughts.

The underlying theme was worry about harm coming to the child. Parents worried that they might be responsible for harm, and they worried about the efforts made to prevent that harm. The researchers argued that unwanted, intrusive thoughts lie on a spectrum. Those who reach the clinical threshold of OCD typically have more distressing symptoms that last longer.[2]

PAUSE FOR THOUGHT

Unwanted intrusive thoughts can occur in healthy individuals and may be influenced by public health concerns. These thoughts also tend to increase among those who are pregnant and after the birth of a baby. This happens for various reasons, but mainly because of the added pressure of caring for their child. Clinical studies recognise that among the non-clinical population surveyed, intrusive thoughts are often isolated and infrequent, especially when compared to those with OCD.

In perinatal mental health services, we understand that many mothers and fathers may feel hesitant to share their unwanted intrusive thoughts. They might worry about being seen as 'bad' parents or even as dangerous, which can be really distressing. There's often a concern that if they talk to a health professional about these thoughts, their child could be taken away by social services. Luckily, such involvement is quite rare and usually only happens when there are additional risks, such as substance misuse or domestic violence. Because of these fears, many parents keep their thoughts private and might delay seeking help for years (Edwards & Timmons 2005). As highlighted in the Fairbrother et al. (2021) study, women experiencing OCD during the perinatal period often have intrusive thoughts related to their infant. Sometimes, they might not mention these in questionnaires. They may complete the questionnaire in relation to themselves – in perinatal OCD many have unwanted intrusive thoughts *about the baby's wellbeing*, without concerns about their own wellbeing. We want parents to know they're not alone and that help is available in a supportive, judgement-free environment.

In perinatal OCD, the intrusive thoughts are frequent and disruptive. One might try to downplay or dismiss unwanted thoughts by labelling them as 'normal'. In clinical practice, we understand that the

2 A noted limitation of the study is that only a quarter of participants completed the survey. As their responses were self-reported, this also introduces a bias in choosing what thoughts are disclosed.

issue is not just the presence of intrusive thoughts. The real problem is their obsessive nature – persistent and repetitive throughout the day – causing significant distress. This often leads to a compulsive urge to perform behaviours or rituals in a desperate attempt to reduce the intensity of these thoughts.

Perinatal OCD during a pandemic

Many patients with OCD, especially those who have obsessional fears of contamination, may become fixated on widespread illnesses that have received media attention over the years, such as HIV/AIDS in the early 1990s and the MRSA 'super bug', which, although first identified in the 1960s, gained prominence in the early 2000s. To evaluate the psychosocial impacts of COVID-19 during pregnancy, a team of psychiatrists and behavioural scientists from New York surveyed nearly 5000 women via social media in May 2020 (Mahaffey et al. 2022). As part of the study, they administered OCD screening questionnaires and discovered that clinically significant OCD symptoms were more than twice as prevalent as in pregnant women before the pandemic. However, it was recognised that the situation is complex, as those facing socio-economic disadvantages may encounter greater challenges concerning their mental wellbeing and social isolation compared to the general population. Furthermore, there is a known rise in washing and ordering symptoms, which may reflect the 'nesting' urge to prepare for a baby's arrival towards the end of pregnancy, as well as increased fears of infection during delivery, particularly among first-time mothers.

CHAPTER 2

Perinatal OCD Psychopathology

Few studies thoroughly investigate the specific psychopathology of perinatal OCD.[1] However, several recent research papers shed light on this emerging field, deepening our understanding of the subtleties of OCD that occur during pregnancy and the postnatal period. Some have argued that it may constitute a distinct condition, separate from OCD seen in the general population, characterised by a cluster of symptoms mainly centred on the health and wellbeing of the baby.

THE CASE FOR PERINATAL OCD AS A UNIQUE CONDITION

The most comprehensive work so far is by Starcevic et al. (2020). They carried out a meta-analysis, collecting 14 studies from 1993 to 2016. In summary, they found that the clinical features of OCD during pregnancy and postpartum are relatively distinct, suggesting that perinatal OCD could be a unique condition with specific symptoms. It was recognised that the perinatal period is a vulnerable time for women, characterised by a 'complex interplay of past experiences and current biological, psychological, and social factors', which may trigger the onset or worsening of mental health disorders during this period (Starcevic et al. 2020). They estimated that pregnant or postnatal women are up to twice as likely to develop OCD compared to the

1 Psychopathology is the study of mental illness in terms of their causes, development, course, classification, and treatment.

general population. The current evidence mainly concentrates on the presentation of OCD in the postnatal period rather than during pregnancy. Specifically, there is an increase in infant-focused obsessions, a heightened risk of aggressive OCD thoughts, thoughts of unintentional harm, fears of contamination coupled with washing/cleaning compulsions, and excessive reassurance-seeking.

DISTINGUISHING FEATURES

Abramowitz et al. (2003b) published a detailed study on perinatal OCD, providing an in-depth analysis of intrusive thoughts and neutralising behaviours or rituals. They discovered that women exhibit unique symptoms not commonly seen in perinatal depression or anxiety disorders. Nearly half of women with diagnosed OCD reported intrusive thoughts about harm coming to the baby through accidents, such as dropping the infant, choking or road traffic accidents, or causing death, like sudden infant death syndrome (SIDS). Of those surveyed, 10–15% experienced unwanted intrusive thoughts of harming the infant through screaming, shaking, or slapping, with 5% reporting unwanted sexual thoughts about the baby. Due to the stigma and shame linked to these thoughts, they were probably under-reported.

Neutralising rituals focused on checking behaviours and reassurance-seeking. A significant 72% of women surveyed engaged in self-reassuring thoughts, such as telling themselves it is 'okay' or seeking reassurance from others. Over two-thirds of women exhibited repetitive checking behaviours related to the baby's welfare. Around 60% chose to distract themselves, and about half preferred to rationalise or repress their thoughts. Nearly 50% prayed about their intrusive thoughts or confided in their partner or parent; 40% confided in others outside of immediate family, seeking reassurance. About a quarter actively removed themselves from situations that might trigger unwanted intrusive thoughts. Only 10% reported avoiding the baby, which feels like an underestimate from a clinical perspective. This may reflect how mothers, often the primary carers in the first year of life, are unable to rely on consistent childcare or other family members to take over parental responsibilities. In the next chapter, we will explore the common subthemes of OCD, and how they may present in the perinatal period.

CHAPTER 3

Subthemes of Perinatal OCD

People with OCD often experience symptoms grouped within specific 'themes'. Although anything can become the focus of one's fears and intrusive thoughts, the principles of how it presents remain the same. The fear of unwanted intrusive thoughts of 'X' leads to increased anxiety, which is then alleviated by performing repetitive behaviours, rituals, or compulsions to reduce the anxiety.

In this chapter, I discuss the unique symptoms that can appear during the perinatal period that may not be detected through routine screening or mental health assessments. New themes may emerge, and old themes may resurface. Themes can also change over time, reflecting the life stage and responsibilities at that time. For example, I have encountered patients who struggled with contamination and body-image issues during their teenage years but became preoccupied with fear of accidental harm to their children once they became parents.

In Figure 3.1, I have summarised how themes of OCD symptoms can overlap with one another, and, in the context of OCD occurring during the perinatal period, these themes may blend. For example, someone might have a fear of being 'dirty' from a physical perspective due to fears of contamination, but also 'dirty' from a psychological or moral perspective. These double meanings add complexity to both the detection and management of the condition.

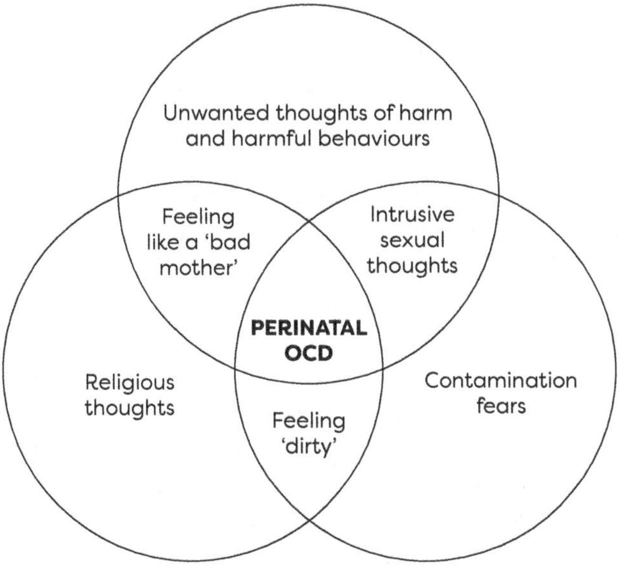

Figure 3.1 How perinatal OCD symptoms overlap

FEAR OF HARM/AGGRESSIVE OCD

Although many people associate OCD with constant cleaning and being a 'neat freak', one of the most common presentations observed involves aggressive and/or violent thoughts. Sufferers have a strong fear that they might harm themselves or others (and in the perinatal setting, 'others' is almost always the baby). People may also experience what I refer to in clinic as a 'flash-forward'. Unlike 'flashbacks' seen in post-traumatic stress disorder (PTSD), they may visualise violent or horrific images of the worst-case scenarios imaginable. Examples patients have described include seeing their children covered in blood by the roadside, convinced they will die in a car crash, or visualising their baby at the bottom of the stairs, scared they may drop them. Other fears are classified as 'aggressive', such as doing or saying something embarrassing, like blurting out vulgar obscenities (similar to Tourette syndrome). There is also a significant fear that something bad might happen and that it will be their fault because they were not careful or responsible enough. This could show in worries about events like a house fire or burglary, where they believe their actions – or inactions – might have prevented the disaster.

As discussed later in the book, anxiety linked to increased responsibility can be especially pronounced for new mothers, who, from conception onwards, face immense societal expectations to be nurturing, responsible, and attentive parents without fault. For those grappling with thoughts of harm or being blamed for mistakes, particularly concerning their own behaviour, the focus of their compulsions is usually on checking actions. Patients often check aspects of the household (stoves, appliances, light switches, locks on windows and doors) multiple times, fearing intruders or harm coming to the family. They may also seek reassurance from themselves and others, checking that they did not or will not harm themselves or others and that nothing terrible has or will happen. This was especially evident when I worked on the inpatient OCD unit. Patients would feel not only the persistent urge to seek reassurance that everything was 'okay' but also a strong need to tell, ask, or confess their thoughts aloud to health professionals.

Terminology differences

A subtle but noticeable difference exists in the terminology used in general OCD compared to perinatal OCD. In general, OCD textbooks commonly refer to thoughts being 'violent' or 'aggressive', whereas in perinatal settings, the wording is softer and passive, following the 'fear of accidental harm' subtheme of OCD. As I discuss in Part 2, I believe this relates to the biases we have about women and mothers in our society, pointing to a collective struggle around accepting that women and mothers may be capable of violent or aggressive thoughts. Although some may argue that they ultimately amount to the same thing, wording is important because it lends itself to disclosure of symptoms (or lack of). Of course, this topic is nuanced, but, given the additional stigma of maternal mental illness (which we discuss more in Part 2), the use of softer language in the perinatal setting is preferred and needed in facilitating patients' seeking help. It is also essential to hold on to the fact that in OCD violent intrusive thoughts do not equate to violent acts. Thus, patients can be reassured with use of appropriate language coupled with psychoeducation.

FEAR OF CONTAMINATION OCD

CASE VIGNETTE – KATIE

I will never forget meeting Katie on the National OCD/BDD Ward. She only had one task that day: to open the door of her bedroom. For most of us, this simple action is completed in a fraction of a second, without a moment's thought.

Opening doors, both physically and metaphorically, enables movement to new places and possibilities. As the saying goes, when one door closes, another opens... but not for Katie. One day, after her therapy session, I found her hiding behind the tall cupboard, her frail, svelte frame wedged between the wall and the back of the heavy oak wardrobe. With the calmest voice, I tried to gently coax her out from behind a cupboard, but Katie would not move. I felt powerless and fragile and imagine this must have been an ounce of what Katie herself was feeling at that time too.

Katie's obsessional beliefs revolved around fear of contamination. Although some would say that this is a typical symptom of OCD, her compulsive behaviours did not reflect the common stereotype.[1] In Katie's case, the fear had paralysed her. She could not begin her morning routine of getting dressed and opening the door to start her day, without the crushing worry that she had contaminated herself by touching the doorknob, or that she had not turned it 'correctly'. She would try starting her morning routine again but continue to fall into the repetitive loop of worry and trying to get it 'just right', which lasted for hours.

Her inability to open the door was not only frustrating but became dangerous. Unable to leave her room, Katie was not engaging with self-care, such as washing, dressing, drinking, or eating. Many patients with severe OCD can develop serious, acute kidney failure because their obsessional thoughts render them unable to perform basic daily tasks and function.

Thankfully, with weeks of intensive, daily psychological therapy in the form of exposure and response prevention (specialised evidence-based cognitive behavioural therapy that is beneficial

1 Despite the wealth of information available, many still believe that someone with OCD 'likes to clean a lot'.

> for OCD patients), alongside medication, Katie was slowly able to open the door, not only of her room, but to the rest of her life, free of debilitating OCD.

Fear of contamination is probably the most well-known symptom associated with OCD. It is much more than simply liking things to be 'clean and tidy' or experiencing the 'nesting' phase in pregnancy, where there is an innate drive to organise the home in preparation for the upcoming arrival. FEAR OF CONTAMINATION OCD involves concerns with bodily waste or secretions, such as urine, faeces, or saliva (often accompanied by the core emotion of disgust). During the perinatal period, this list can expand to include many other secretions, including breast milk, sperm, ejaculate, vaginal discharge, blood, and vomit. Fears may involve environmental and biological contaminants, such as soil, dirt, radiation, and toxins like asbestos, and the risks they pose. Other contamination fears may relate to bacterial or viral infections and communicable diseases, such as HIV/AIDS.

Pregnancy is a very uncertain time for mothers, as they feel the added burden of being 100% responsible for the wellbeing of the foetus. Patients may present with concerns that reflect current news items, fearing that they have been exposed to the featured illness or contamination. Anxiety related to the real and/or perceived risk of contracting illnesses during pregnancy that could affect the baby (NHS 2024) is particularly important to be aware of. Typical examples include COVID-19, Zika virus, rubella, or chickenpox. Additional risks in pregnancy from animal or food-related contamination may also present as obsessions.[2]

After delivery, fears of contamination may extend to the baby, especially regarding the child becoming ill from 'infected' breast milk, contaminated formula, or germs left on bottles. To address this, a parent might avoid breastfeeding altogether or develop compulsive routines such as repeatedly cleaning bottles or checking ingredients on formula packaging. In FEAR OF CONTAMINATION OCD, the mother often seeks full control to be '100% sure' that there is no risk to their

2 Risks in pregnancy include contracting toxoplasmosis (from cat faeces) and, based on new evidence, possible hepatitis E infection from close contact with sheep.

baby. Family members may want to assist with the demanding, repetitive tasks or feeding routines, but the person with OCD may be hesitant to relinquish control due to fear that their partner, mother, or in-laws will 'do it wrong', which can increase their anxiety and lead to doing 'double work'.

Parents might also feel anxious about friends or family members touching or kissing their newborn, or the baby being 'passed around' at social gatherings. Naturally, this feeling is quite common among new mothers, especially since the COVID-19 pandemic and before their newborn is fully immunised. However, it is important to consider the threshold for OCD – a condition that can significantly impact quality of life and daily activities. It can harm relationships, leading to avoidance of people or places that might trigger heightened anxiety or unwanted intrusive thoughts. Consequently, those with the condition may steer clear of unfamiliar environments or focus more on completing compulsive rituals at home.

For those who have fears of contamination, the response often involves compulsive and excessive cleaning of themselves and their homes. During the postnatal period, their compulsive behaviours may extend to their children. Patients frequently describe highly ritualised and detailed routines of hand washing, showering, bathing, grooming, and using the toilet, which must be performed repeatedly throughout the day, especially if they leave the house or see someone outside their immediate family. Clinicians may also notice common themes of order, symmetry, and a need for 'exactness'. For instance, each body part might be washed in a specific way (e.g. clockwise or counterclockwise), or for a set number of times, before moving on to the next. If interrupted or if they feel they have not done it 'correctly', they often feel compelled to start again. I have encountered women who washed their hands so frequently that they became dry, cracked, and raw, necessitating urgent referral to dermatology.

This behaviour is not only time-consuming but also emotionally and physically exhausting for both the person with OCD and their family, who are often subjected to strict cleanliness routines. The danger from this behaviour is both physical and social. Parents may become socially avoidant out of fear of contamination (including parent–baby groups groups), and OCD can interfere with schooling needs and healthcare appointments. Patients may force their children to be washed 'head to toe' on their return from school. Without intervention, such behaviour can infringe on child rights and safety, potentially leading to further assessment of the child's welfare by social care in extreme cases.

Mental contamination

There has been recent research on the concept of 'mental contamination'. This can occur when an individual feels overly criticised, judged, or mistreated on a personal level (alluding to the common phrase 'made me feel like dirt'). Mental contamination almost always comes from human contact (as opposed to inanimate objects or external hazards); however, it does not require physical proximity with others to occur (Mind 2023). It is important in the clinical setting to make the distinction between thoughts being 'contaminated' and paranoid ideation, which is often seen in delusional disorders and schizophrenia. This critical differential diagnosis is discussed in greater detail in Chapter 13.

RELIGIOUS OCD (SCRUPULOSITY)

CASE VIGNETTE – YASMIN

I met Yasmin at the start of her first pregnancy when she was 26 years old. I will never forget her because she arrived at her first appointment carrying her diary with a detailed account of her journey with OCD. She noted that it began when she was a young child, with a preoccupation with death and dying.

Yasmin grew up in Egypt, and her family are devout Muslims. From a young age, she associated cleanliness with purity. She remembers that her OCD symptoms worsened when she became a teenager. Around this time, her grandmother explained to her the importance of cleanliness in their Islamic faith and gave her instructions for personal hygiene rituals, especially around her monthly menstruation. When on her period during Ramadan, she was exempt from fasting but was encouraged to 'make up for it' afterwards with additional fasting and prayers.

Yasmin described feeling 'obsessed' with being a 'good, moral person' since her teenage years. When she started working, she would allocate a significant portion of her salary to charity, prioritising these donations over her regular bills and rent. She also noted that her fears about being 'impure' or 'sinful' affected her ability to form relationships. Only in recent years, after moving away from her strict family upbringing to study abroad, was she able to release some of the guilt and shame she had felt in childhood.

Yasmin told me that she had seen many psychiatrists and been prescribed various medications, including potent antipsychotics. However, it was only after our assessment confirming OCD and having accessed psychological therapy and the appropriate medications for her condition that she finally felt 'free' of her mental illness. This liberation gave her the mental space and energy to enjoy motherhood.

RELIGIOUS OCD, also known as 'SCRUPULOSITY', is a type of OCD that centres around worries related to religious and spiritual thoughts, images, and actions. People with this condition often fret over doing or saying things they believe might be wrong, immoral, or not aligned with their faith. They might worry about committing blasphemy (speech or actions perceived as showing disrespect to God or a deity) or about offending God or sacred places of worship. Often, they hold beliefs that they are 'a bad person', 'sinful', or that they are 'going to hell'. They may also become obsessive about aspects of their spiritual practices, like fearing they are not praying 'correctly' or wearing the hijab the right way. Similar to concerns about contamination during the perinatal period, these intrusive thoughts can sometimes extend to their infants, with worries that the baby might be 'unholy' because of the parents' faults, or preoccupations with baptism, religious ceremonies, or excessive praying for their children.

Compulsive behaviours in relation to SCRUPULOSITY include:

- praying frequently and obsessively (more than what would be considered 'normal' in one's religion)
- excessive, repetitive counting of prayer beads or time-consuming religious customs and rituals

- a constant urge to confess one's sins
- doing altruistic acts in the hope that it proves they are a 'good' person
- avoiding places that may trigger feelings of immorality
- avoiding intimacy.

This type of OCD is more prevalent in regions where strict religious and cultural norms are present, such as the Middle East. It is also more widespread among individuals raised in strict religious environments, especially within the Muslim or Catholic faiths (Abramowitz & Jacoby 2014).

For those with RELIGIOUS OCD, as with all OCD subthemes, obsessional thoughts and rituals are not pleasurable. Instead, they cause intense fear, distress, and worry. Rather than finding comfort in their faith or spiritual practice, people often feel burdened by their thoughts and experience significant guilt and shame. As I will discuss in Part 2, when seen in perinatal OCD, this phenomenon frequently overlaps with maternal guilt and shame related to not feeling 'good enough'.

Yasmin's experience illustrates how cultural and familial factors significantly influence RELIGIOUS OCD. The boundaries between adherence to moral or religious teachings, feelings of shame, and mental health stigma are often unclear. In such cases, family therapy can be helpful in exploring some of the beliefs and 'family scripts' that were taught or believed as a child and continue to be held as an adult. Some individuals with OCD may not have a religious background but find comfort within a religious setting, which 'permits' or even celebrates their obsessions and compulsions as signs of being 'devout' followers.[3]

ORDER/SYMMETRY OCD

CASE VIGNETTE – SAM

One of my first experiences in mental health was working on an inpatient psychiatric unit. For many people in this field, it feels like

3 For more on RELIGIOUS OCD, see https://iocdf.org

a 'rite of passage' because you encounter some of the most unwell individuals. Learning about psychiatric diagnoses and treatments can be quite a steep journey, but it really lays a strong foundation for working in community settings and handling crisis situations.

I will never forget meeting Sam. It was around 5pm, just as handover was taking place. I was the doctor on the 'long day' shift until 9pm and was being updated on the jobs to be passed on to me. Sam had been admitted that afternoon. The day team informed me that they were causing quite a stir on the ward, appearing quite unwell and preoccupied, which made it difficult to have a proper conversation with them.

I didn't quite understand what the day team meant until I saw Sam for myself. They were standing in the communal corridor outside the nurses' station, looking quite agitated and restless. They had laid all their books and other personal items they had brought to the ward – such as a hairbrush, toothbrush, jumper, and birthday card – on the floor, arranging them in a row, stretching from one end of the corridor to the other.

Sam spent a lot of time adjusting them to make sure they were 'perfectly symmetrical'. They then became flustered and tried to organise them by size, placing the biggest books at the far end of the corridor and working their way down to the smallest items closer to their feet.

Other patients, each dealing with their own illnesses, were walking around, equally bewildered by this seemingly strange behaviour. Some were watching, while others were chuckling quietly to themselves. I could see Sam becoming more and more upset because they felt they couldn't get it 'right'. A few patients were growing annoyed as they felt Sam's actions were disrupting the ward routine. The books were blocking the door to the dining room, and Sam wouldn't let anyone step over them, worried about bringing bad luck.

Order- and symmetry-based obsessions are quite common in OCD within community settings. However, we rarely see them emerge acutely on inpatient wards, as they often 'flourish' within the controlled environment of a home. As the name suggests, preoccupations involve obsessional thoughts and images centred on items being 'in order'. Symmetry obsessions are characterised by the need for things to be perfect, exact, or 'just right', aligned correctly, and in a balanced way. The need for symmetry may also relate to mathematical concepts such as Pythagorean theory, geometrical design, and obsession with shapes, spirals, and tessellations. Another aspect involves mirroring, which is observed both in nature and in concerns around facial symmetry, facial features, body symmetry, and the external appearance of oneself and others.

Related compulsions include ordering and arranging, evening up or aligning objects, and touching or tapping. This is usually coupled with intense feelings of distress when things are not 'perfectly aligned'. Although on the surface one might assume that this subtheme of OCD is less serious, research shows that OCD patients with primary symmetry-related symptoms had significantly higher OCD severity scores, longer illness durations, and increased psychiatric comorbidity, including risk of self-harm (in the absence of childhood trauma or triggers). This suggests that the presence of primary symmetry-related symptoms may serve as a marker of severity in OCD (Lochner et al. 2016).

In perinatal OCD, the risk is extending the need for perfect order to the baby, as generally, the postnatal period with a baby is anything but orderly. The lack of control, routine, or time to match things exactly (such as folding muslin cloths precisely), or the potential for a baby to 'ruin' the symmetry of the building blocks they are playing with, for example, can cause significant distress to mothers with ORDER/SYMMETRY OCD.

SEXUAL/RELATIONSHIP OCD

Sexual obsessions are quite common among those experiencing perinatal OCD, but they are rarely reported compared to other symptoms. These include unwanted intrusive thoughts that the individual believes are 'forbidden', or visualising unwanted graphic images. The content of these thoughts is often considered wrong in the mind of the person or frowned upon in their culture (especially if they were raised in a strict and/or religious family) and in wider society.

Examples include intrusive and distressing thoughts about homosexuality, bestiality, incest, and non-consensual sexual behaviours towards others. In perinatal OCD, these thoughts may focus on babies and children, with fears of being a paedophile (or that people perceive them to be a paedophile) or that they are/have been perpetrators of sexual abuse (Chaudhary, Singh, & Varshney 2022).

Given the intimate nature of a parent–child relationship, which involves responsibilities such as feeding, bathing, and clothing young children, the perinatal period can be a triggering time for both mothers and fathers experiencing OCD. Mothers may avoid breastfeeding by choosing formula feeding, out of fear they will experience erotic urges, thoughts, or images while the baby is sucking on their nipple. Sex and breastfeeding share biological similarities, as the 'love' hormone oxytocin is released during both orgasm and lactation. Others may find being in close contact with the baby's genital areas (such as when changing a nappy) difficult, as it may trigger unwanted thoughts or images.

SEXUAL/RELATIONSHIP OCD is an emerging subtheme of OCD. It can present in various forms, including fears centred on a partner, usually the person's romantic partner. It can present in various forms, including excessive doubt about the relationship, extending to concerns about fidelity. In perinatal OCD, I have encountered this subtheme much more often than in my non-perinatal OCD patients. A common presentation is an expectant mother who arranges multiple DNA tests to confirm whether her partner is the father of the child, due to unwanted, intrusive thoughts about whether she has had sexual intercourse with someone else. This fear leads to high levels of anxiety, and the compulsive checking for 'proof' temporarily alleviates the anxiety. If disclosed, these fears often require a lot of reassurance, which can strain the relationship.

In these circumstances, it is important to ensure that all other possible explanations for the presentation have been explored. First, investigate whether the doubts may reflect a truth regarding undisclosed infidelity. One must also check for any safeguarding concerns regarding alleged sexual assaults or past trauma of childhood sexual abuse. Clinicians should be mindful of concerns during a patient's pregnancy or with the development of the foetus, including possible overlapping fears of contamination surrounding sexually transmitted infections coupled with infidelity.

'Pure O'

The purely obsessional (or, as some call it, 'Pure O') subtheme of OCD is something I didn't encounter much until I started working with women in the perinatal period. Although the empirical evidence to date is limited, its main symptom is intrusive obsessional thoughts, without the ritualistic compulsive behaviours that usually accompany it.

'Pure O' can manifest in various ways. One distinctive presentation I have observed during the perinatal period involves obsessional fears about the patient's partner, with significant doubts arising regarding whether that person is the father of the unborn child. Some may also categorise this as 'relational OCD', as the focus is on the relationship or partner dynamic. Many individuals, however, do not view reassurance-seeking as 'compulsive', but rather as a natural instinct to navigate and confirm their obsessional thoughts. Consequently, 'pure OCD' remains a debated issue within clinical and research circles, yet it continues to be a prominent concept among patients and in OCD/parenting support forums.

CASE VIGNETTE – SALLY: RELATIONAL OCD OR PURE O?

Sally was 24 years old and expecting her first child with her partner, Ben. They were engaged to be married after a three-year relationship, but they had known each other since secondary school. Ben seemed to be a loyal and caring fiancé. He attended all her antenatal appointments, and Sally said she had no concerns about their relationship. The pregnancy, although unplanned, was welcomed.

Sally was referred to perinatal mental health services by her midwife during the final trimester of her pregnancy because she was feeling 'anxious about the pregnancy'. As with many referrals to perinatal mental health services, the initial reason often only scratches the surface, and it is only through further assessment that the real issues are revealed. Sally confided in me that she

> couldn't shake the thought that Ben was not the father of her child. When I asked her to elaborate, she mentioned that she had never been unfaithful and had no reason to suspect he had been, but for some reason she couldn't get the idea out of her mind – this idea came in the form of unwanted intrusive thoughts.
>
> Sally had also arranged for multiple privately funded DNA tests without Ben's knowledge to confirm if he was indeed the father. Although each test confirmed his paternity, she never felt truly satisfied with the results and would begin organising another. She said her intrusive thoughts worsened as her pregnancy progressed; any unrelated man she encountered during the day (such as the bus driver or postman) would trigger beliefs that he was the father of her unborn child.
>
> Sally told me that she knew she 'sounded crazy' because there was no way anyone else could be the father of her child. She was in a monogamous relationship and had never met these other men, let alone had intimate encounters with them. According to Ben, Sally would ask him at least ten times a day for reassurance that he was the father. And he would offer that reassurance, as he felt it was the 'right thing to do to ease her mind'. It became somewhat awkward when I was asked how many times is 'too many' to reassure someone. Yet, this is the million-dollar question.

In the case of OCD, it's often felt that no matter how much is offered, it's never quite enough. The urge to seek reassurance just never truly satisfies. We also understand that seeking reassurance can be a significant challenge for families and partners, placing a heavy strain on them. They often find themselves in a difficult position, living with someone caught up in the depths of intrusive thoughts, where reassurance appears to be the only source of comfort and temporary peace.

On the surface, Sally appears to have a purely obsessional subtheme of OCD, characterised by unwelcome intrusive thoughts of infidelity. Some might argue that the reassurance-seeking behaviours (such as repeatedly 'checking in' with her partner and the DNA tests) could actually be regarded as compulsive actions, thus fulfilling the criteria for OCD.

MISCELLANEOUS/SOMATIC OCD

This form of OCD does not fit into a neat 'theme' but can be just as limiting and challenging to deal with. Almost anything can become a focus in OCD. With this in mind, we don't fixate on specific symptoms but rather on:

- general principles of the obsessions that cause a feeling of anxiety
- compulsions as an attempt to neutralise the fear
- a pattern of thoughts and behaviour that repeats numerous times a day.

In MISCELLANEOUS/SOMATIC OCD, the obsessions focus on concepts such as needing to know or remember things, fear of saying or thinking certain things, and fear of not saying the 'right' thing. There may also be repetitive, intrusive images of a non-violent nature, as well as nonsense words, sounds, or music. Those with this type of OCD may also be sensitive to superstitious fears, with preferences for certain colours, lucky or unlucky numbers, odd or even numbers, or a compulsion to count a specific number of times to their 'lucky number', either in their head or out loud. Other common compulsions include mental rituals (such as checking, counting, or excessive list-making), vocal rituals (needing to tell, ask, or 'confess' their thoughts), or physical rituals (touching, tapping, blinking, pinching, or rubbing themselves or measuring things). Some describe this OCD as 'somatic' because of bodily preoccupations in obsessive thoughts and compulsive routines, along with concerns about illness, disease, or appearance. These symptoms can affect all aspects of daily life, including eating, hygiene, and sleeping routines.

At its most severe, it can impair quality of life and daily functioning as someone becomes 'stuck' in their routine, unable to move forward until things are 'correct'. With somatic and/or miscellaneous OCD, there is significant overlap with other types of OCD (e.g. RELIGIOUS OCD, ORDER/SYMMETRY OCD) as well as related disorders (e.g. body dysmorphic disorder, health anxiety, and trichotillomania). In the perinatal period, it is especially challenging as it consumes time, a scarce resource during the postnatal phase. They might experience heightened anxiety and/or frustration with themselves if unable to complete their tasks. They may perceive the baby's needs as 'competing' for their time, or feel too distracted, overwhelmed, or exhausted to manage the daily tasks of raising a child, often requiring substantial support from others.

To reassure or not to reassure, that is the question

One of the most common questions I get from staff, patients, and families alike is whether to reassure the person with OCD or not, and if so, how often is too often. The hallmark of OCD in all its forms is that nothing is ever enough. A person may clean their house from top to bottom but still feel unsatisfied. They worry that one cough will throw everything into disarray and cause contamination, meaning they'll need to start the cleaning process all over again.

Reassurance-seeking is similar. Those who have experienced it will know all too well that it is never 'just once'. The reassurance may not only relate to the OCD but also to the relationship, such as asking repeatedly 'Do you love me?' or 'Do you hate me?' Those requesting reassurance or checking will do so multiple times a day, which can place a significant strain on relationships. Initial empathy for a partner or friend can spiral into irritation, anger, avoidance, or resentment. One can oscillate between offering too much reassurance and none at all.

'Blocking' reassurance may only make things worse in the immediate period. Individuals may become very upset and agitated and/or find other unhealthy ways to neutralise their anxiety. Rather than 'being cruel to be kind', it can be extremely distressing for the individual with OCD.

For those living with a person with OCD, reassurance-seeking can make home life intolerable. Often, family members will collude with the individual to 'keep the peace'. This may occur especially when a new baby has arrived. A mother will constantly ask her partner or mother to help with checking behaviours around the house, and everyone will oblige, as it can be difficult to know how to resist supporting this compulsive checking, which, on the surface, is viewed as 'the right thing to do' to ensure the baby's safety.

The UK charity OCD Action advises against focusing on OCD itself and the vicious cycle of reassurance-seeking and instead recommends concentrating on the relationship. The aim is not to stop reassurance abruptly but to support the person in making a conscious decision to reduce and eventually cease seeking reassurance. As the condition can completely take over a person's life, it is important to attempt to recover some of the lost aspects of the relationship.

Those living with a person with OCD can support them by:

- finding things to do together outside of the cycle of reassurance-seeking
- acknowledging the request for reassurance, as this itself can be reassuring and is a healthy way to show support
- finding other mutual ways to reduce the moment of anxiety together, such as making a cup of tea, giving a hug, or going for a walk for some fresh air with the baby in the pram
- reassuring in the moment to move the day forward if the situation is acute and feels 'stuck'; 'go along' and provide the reassurance to avoid a serious incident, but consider bringing the topic back at a moment of calm where you and the person with OCD can talk about ways to manage future escalations, creating a joint 'care plan'
- encouraging the person with OCD to discuss the behaviour with their therapist, if the person is in therapy, or indeed having a joint session with their loved one on how best to manage the topic of reassurance; this issue can cause difficulties within a relationship, so it can be helpful to have someone objective and 'outside' of the family to help navigate tough conversations.

RECOVERY

Despite the range and extent of distressing themes experienced in perinatal OCD, the important thing is that recovery is possible. Recognising its presentation allows for a diagnosis and access to treatment options. Through perinatal mental health support, psychological therapy, or medication (which we discuss later in Part 5 of the book), women can regain control of their health and wellbeing and enjoy motherhood without the constraints of the illness. Motherhood, however, is not without its challenges. In Part 2, we will explore in greater depth the impact motherhood has on OCD and mental health, and how our biological and social programming can intensify the experiences of perinatal OCD. I also dedicate a chapter to the anatomy of perfectionism and its complex relationship with OCD during the perinatal period.

PART 2

MOTHERHOOD, OCD, AND MENTAL HEALTH

The transition to motherhood, known as 'matrescence', is, without a doubt, one of the most significant life events an individual can experience. She has changed not only on a biological level, but also emotionally, psychologically, socially, hormonally, and physically. When a child is born, a mother is also born. A new identity is created in her and will remain with her however old her 'children' become. Although she may find herself alone, she is kept company by not only her children, but the ideas and expectations built through her life experiences on what a mother should (and should not) be. These beliefs may stem from the way she was parented by her own mother, the individual for whom most of us is our main reference on how to 'be' (or not to be) a mother.

There are, of course, other sources of powerful inspiration and information, from other maternal figures in our lives (whether they be related or not), as well as our collective societal ideation of motherhood, or should I say idealisation of motherhood. As esteemed writer and forensic psychotherapist Estela Welldon describes in her seminal book *Mother, Madonna, Whore: The Idealisation and Denigration of Motherhood*, mothers are often given a 'Madonna' complex – innocence and virtuosity personified, free of blame or wrong (Welldon 1992). Of course, women and mothers are far from perfect. Throughout time, women and mothers have been held to stratospheric heights of expectation, both externally by others but also internally instilled, striving for perfection in their work, home, and appearance.

Our current generation, as well as those that follow, face the added stressor of comparison being readily available online, 24 hours a day, seven days a week. Friends and virtual strangers candidly detail every aspect of their motherhood experience with a highlight reel of blossoming careers, clutter-free homes, and well-behaved children. Even for those that vow to 'keep it real', there is often a subtle sense of a filtered lens, where the thief of joy is all too palpable. To fully understand perinatal OCD, we first need to grasp the nuances of the transition into motherhood and the individual, cultural, and societal expectations placed on expectant mothers to be perfect. Additionally, we must consider how this pursuit of perfection aligns with beliefs surrounding maternal wellness and illness in perinatal OCD (Pedrucci 2020).

The second part of this book focuses on the maternal mind. Chapter 4 examines the concept of motherhood and maternal identity, exploring the intersection of nurture and nature by discussing the science behind maternal instincts and the historical assignment of the primary caregiving role to women. In Chapter 5, I analyse perfectionism in detail, including the ideas, expectations, and difficulties that can arise throughout the perinatal journey, from fertility and pregnancy to parenting. I explore the notion of being a 'good enough mother' and consider how OCD and perfectionism raise questions like 'what if good enough isn't good enough?' The final chapter of Part 2 addresses the specific challenges that OCD, especially perinatal OCD, can present – how it may affect the journey to becoming pregnant, as well as its impact on one's own sense of self and relationships within the family. We conclude Chapter 6 with the 'three Ps' of OCD and motherhood: a helpful aide-mémoire to understand the shared commonalities of OCD and motherhood, and the difficulties that may arise when either one is dysregulated.

CHAPTER 4

Ideas of Motherhood – Nurture Meets Nature

In this chapter, we will explore the historical aspects of womanhood and how they shape our expectations and understanding of motherhood in the 21st century, as well as how this has been depicted in the creative arts on stage and in film. As discussed in Part 1, the evolution of OCD as a clinical condition is a complex journey, influenced by societal pressures and practices of different eras. Similarly, our understanding of becoming a mother – or what it means to be a 'good' or 'bad' mother – is largely influenced by preconceived ideas. I will also briefly examine our biological understanding of maternal love, as well as how motherhood is portrayed in modern society.

THE 'DOMESTIC GODDESS'

Historically, 'mother' has been a loaded term, filled with rich symbolism in art, literature, and religion. From Madonna, the mother of Christ, to Gaia, the mother of Earth, the maternal is universally seen as a loving and nurturing female quality. For many, simply thinking of the term 'mother' can evoke a visceral response of caring and feelings of selfless love (Pedrucci 2020). In contrast, the term 'father' does not carry the same high standards and expectations associated with caring for children. Instead, it conveys a sense of responsibility, often linked to protective authority. This is clear in its use in Christianity, especially in patriarchal references to God, as in the common opening and closing liturgy for prayer: 'In the name of the Father, the Son, and the Holy Spirit'.

This prerequisite of the 'mother' being a loving, nurturing presence formed the foundation of family law in the 1800s. Although mothers were responsible for childcare (included as part of their domestic duties), they had very little influence in terms of actual financial or social power. They were viewed as the inferior parent compared to fathers, who were not only the breadwinners but also the head of the household, making all the crucial decisions. Gradually, however, there was a gentle shift away from patriarchy towards prioritising the wellbeing of children. The Tender Years Doctrine, a legal principle in English family law from the 19th century, embodied the symbolism of the loving, nurturing mother. It endorsed the widely held societal belief that it was in a child's best interest to be in the custody of the mother during the 'tender years' (age four and under). Some have argued that this laid the groundwork for the expectation that a woman's place was in the home, excluding women from paid work, under the patriarchal guise of protecting and sheltering women to help them reach their 'true potential' as childrearers (Ashraf & Jepsen 2024).

From the 20th century onwards, the analysis of motherhood began to take a darker turn. The goddess-like maternal figure once revered started to diminish and became a focus for blame, not only for the ills of her children but also for wider societal issues. Judgement also began to emerge regarding the quality of mothering, where the term 'unfit' mother was used to describe mothers who engaged in sexual behaviours such as adultery, cohabitation, and sexual orientation. We now know that these behaviours have no bearing on one's ability to be a fit parent (Fineman 1992).

Mothers at the movies

The acclaimed British film director Alfred Hitchcock introduces the concept of the 'difficult mother' in many of his movies, possibly a projection of his reportedly strained relationship with his own mother, and the societal views of mothers at the time. He depicts these matriarchal figures as controlling, intrusive, and domineering – a stark contrast to the sexy blonde bombshell women who often appear alongside his leading men. Films such as *Marnie*, *Rebecca*, and *The Man Who Knew Too Much* all depict a problematic maternal figure with a negative influence. The film *Psycho*, released in 1960, arguably Hitchcock's most famous work and frequently regarded as one of the greatest films of all time, focuses on themes of motherhood and mental health. Norman Bates has a delicate yet pathological relationship with his mother – he famously describes that 'a mother is a son's best friend', but this quote is bittersweet, knowing that analysts and psychiatrists interpret the character, played masterfully by Tony Perkins, as having a dissociative disorder or multiple personality disorder. The portrayal suggests that his mother's cruel and abusive treatment towards him as a child contributed, to some extent, to his violent behaviour later in life.[1]

The idealised notion of motherhood is also questioned as mothers, thinkers, and writers begin to adopt a narrative that diverges from the traditional image of the doting homemaker accepting her husband's and children's authority. In the play *A Doll's House*, written by Norwegian playwright Henrik Ibsen in 1879, the audience was so shocked by the ending (spoiler alert: that the mother chooses to leave her husband and children to pursue an independent life) that it had to be rewritten and performed again with a more socially acceptable ending.

Simone de Beauvoir, a critical feminist, noted that high expectations and self-sacrifice lead to 'inferior mothering', both for the mother and the child. She argues that marriage and children create a culture of obligation and intimacy, designed to keep women from the progressive culture of independence and autonomy (de Beauvoir 1949/2015). Professor Amia Srinivasan, Chichele Professor of Social and Political Theory at the University of Oxford, takes feminist theory and philosophy a step further in her collection of essays *The Right to Sex? Feminist Theory in the 21st Century*. In the essay 'Sex, Carceralism and Capitalism', she dissects the idea of what a woman's 'work' is – work, housework, and sex work – and the boundaries placed upon women not only to perform but also to be perfect in all areas of their lives (Srinivasan 2021).

1 For a discussion of women in Hitchcock films, see Modleski (2015).

Although we know that perinatal OCD is so much more than being 'the perfect mother', we also are aware that for many, the core fears are in relation to its opposite – being the imperfect mother or being deemed as a failure through making a mistake or being responsible for something terrible happening.

Mother knows best

The 2010 Disney animated film *Tangled* is an adaptation of the classic fairy tale of Rapunzel. In the film, the Witch keeps Rapunzel locked away in the tower under the guise of protecting her, while actually using control to assert her authority – a theme expressed in the song 'Mother Knows Best'. The song and the relationship between the Witch and Rapunzel made me reflect on the complexities of the mother–child relationship, especially in cases of perinatal OCD, where 'fear of harm' is the main symptom. If we examine the meaning of the word 'tangle' further, we might see it as something woven, but there is a fine line between something that is intricately woven together (like the bond between a mother and child) and one that is tangled, enmeshed, and impossible to separate, which can also reflect the mother–child relationship. As every parent understands, there is a delicate balance between protecting our children and overprotecting them. It is natural to want the best for them and to do everything possible to prevent harm. Of course, newborns are indeed entirely dependent on their parents for every need. However, even in the first year, we begin to notice significant changes in the infant as they start to develop a sense of self and recognise that they indeed exist independently from their mother. Even in the simple act of watching a baby take their first tentative steps, parents observe closely with concern that the child may fall and hurt themselves. As parents, one naturally clears the path to ensure there are no hazards nearby that the child might trip over. However, as much as one tries to control the environment, the truth remains that in those first important steps, the baby will stumble and then get back up to try again. It can be quite difficult for a caring mother to step back as her child takes a few steps forward. It is a subtle yet significant learning curve in parenting to allow our children to figure things out for themselves, which includes making mistakes along the way.

In perinatal OCD, a lot of time and effort can be spent attempting to control or influence certain factors to reduce the risk of harm; however, it is impossible to control every variable. It may seem easier and safer to settle for being locked away in our own tower to avoid the dangers of the unknown outside. Avoidance plays a significant role in perinatal OCD, and many parents struggling with this condition choose to avoid certain situations or environments (such as family gatherings, parent–baby groups, or public spaces like playgrounds and libraries), preferring to stay at home out of fear of harm to the child or exposure to contamination. As one patient told me, 'My dirt [at home] is different from outside dirt, it's safe.' Symptoms of perinatal OCD can overlap with traits of perfectionism; however, we recognise in both clinical practice and scientific research that there is no such thing as perfection – at best, it is just an illusion or, should I say, a fairy tale.

A MOTHER'S LOVE

Neurobiologist Semir Zeki's paper on the neurobiology of love examines the components of love, including romantic and maternal love, recognising that love is vital for the evolution of the species (Zeki 2007). In his research study on maternal love, he notes that there is activation of 'the love hormones' oxytocin and vasopressin, which in turn deactivate areas of the brain associated with producing negative emotions or judging others. This may, in part, explain why new parents often show no qualms about making silly faces or speaking 'babyese' to entertain their babies in public – a behaviour that would be considered awkward and embarrassing without the presence of a child! Zeki notes an increase in dopamine, the key hormone in the reward mechanism and heavily involved in the 'feel good' sensation of being addicted. A decrease in serotonin is also observed, which is linked to appetite and mood.

OCD also involves a similar depletion of serotonin, and Zeki links the two by stating that 'love, after all, is a kind of obsession', especially in the early stage of falling in love, where there is intense preoccupation and focus on the new partner in romantic love, or the mother 'obsessed' with her newborn. Nerve growth factor (NGF) is another chemical released from the mid-brain, responsible for the initial 'head over heels' rush of hormones whilst falling in love (Esch & Stefano 2005).

Vasopressin and oxytocin are the core hormones responsible for attachment and bonding. They are produced in the hypothalamus and released into the bloodstream, peaking during orgasm and lactation. What is also quite fascinating is that specific areas of the brain involved in feelings of maternal love, attachment, and bonding only become activated when mothers view pictures of their own children, as opposed to other children unknown to them (Cohen, Maroun, & Wagner 2018). This confirms much of our understanding about the special relationship between a parent and child, which from the time of birth is mutually rewarding and desired by both parties. Fascinatingly, many of the brain areas identified as dominant in patients with OCD also play a leading role in maternal sensitivity, bonding, and attachment. The basal ganglia, orbitofrontal cortex, and thalamus have all been found to have increased activity in positive maternal–child attachment (Martínez-García et al. 2021). This undeniable overlap between a healthy maternal love, first-time parent anxiety, and maternal OCD may make clinical sense, even though there are currently no research studies to prove this hypothesis.

Functional magnetic resonance imaging (fMRI) opened the door to a better understanding of the neurobiological basis of human behaviour and experience. In 1999, Lorberbaum et al. reported the responses of four mothers to infants crying, and that small study became the cornerstone of a specialised area of research into understanding maternal bonding and attachment. It sought biological explanations for what we already know well from a psychodynamic perspective – that a mother's love is not only unique but also critical for healthy child development, and a lack of it can have disastrous and even dangerous consequences.

Despite this pioneering research, a recent meta-analysis revealed that over the past two decades only a handful of studies worldwide have explored the neurobiology of maternal love, involving only 147 participants – involving between 6 and 30 per study. Most samples are too small to draw clinically useful conclusions (Shih et al. 2022). While further research is essential, the early data can still help enhance our understanding of the neurobiology of maternal love, offering insights into perinatal OCD.

MATERNAL INSTINCTS

Whenever I hear the phrase 'Mama Bear', it immediately evokes the image of a larger, protective mother who would do anything for her babies. But the latest scientific evidence isn't about bears, but mice. Several studies have examined the behaviour of mice around their offspring. A recent Californian study found that female mice adjust their behaviour before and after giving birth – making themselves sexually approachable prior to their first impregnation but attacking male mice when lactating to protect the baby mice. After pups are weaned, the mothers develop maternal aggressiveness, yet they can switch between sexual advances and resistance to protect pups from infanticide. These changes are believed to occur at a cellular level, through oestrogen-specific neurones in the brain, thereby displaying a 'mama mouse' instinct (Liu et al. 2022).

Another study in mice examined not only the quality but also the quantity of maternal interactions. As expected, if a mother is physically separated from her pup for extended periods during early life, it can trigger acute stress in both the mother and the pup. The quality of care, however, also causes chronic stress. When maternal mice were kept with their pups inside the cage but with home comforts removed (such as the nest providing warmth and protection), it resulted in erratic behaviours and fragmented maternal care towards their pups (Korosi & Baram 2009). The study goes on to demonstrate that mothers, although physically present, can be psychologically or emotionally absent in a child's life. Exposure to external stressors such as war, famine, poverty, drug abuse, or mental illness can influence maternal behaviour. This can have long-lasting effects on children, affecting their cognitive development and their vulnerability or resilience to mental health issues later in life.

Although there are no specific studies examining this phenomenon among mothers with OCD, one can imagine that the time and energy spent adhering to intrusive obsessional thoughts and compulsive behaviours may lead to chronic stress and anxiety, affecting the quality and quantity of time spent with the infant. Although she may be present, OCD symptoms can be distracting, and, if left untreated, all-consuming. One thing I have been told by many mothers with perinatal OCD is that managing OCD is exhausting and draining, partly due to the mental effort required to protect their children and others from the burden of their obsessive ruminations and compulsive rituals. That said, I have seen many mothers in clinical practice who work very hard to protect the bond and attachment with their baby to ensure that OCD does not interfere with their relationship and to minimise the impact on themselves as much as possible.

THE SOCIALISATION INTO MOTHERHOOD

When my youngest daughter was born, I noticed a significant change in her elder sister's attitudes, behaviours, and interests. At not even two years old, it seemed like an internal maternal 'switch' had flipped. While I cared for the newborn, she sat beside me, caring for 'baby Teddy' – changing his nappies, pushing him in his pram to put him to sleep, and even lifting her shirt to proudly 'breastfeed' him. I know much of this imitation came from observing us introduce the new family member, but I couldn't help but wonder how these actions appeared so instinctive to her. Although we gently stopped her from poking her sister during their first meeting, we didn't force her to be caring or tell her this is what girls do. Over time, I saw her embracing her femininity more – our lives now revolve around frilly dresses, Disney princesses, and, as cliché as it sounds, the colour pink.

There are several sociological and feminist studies that explore this in more detail, especially how young girls are socialised to learn about motherhood. Sociologist Ann Oakley even suggests that, unlike in the animal kingdom, there is no maternal instinct, arguing that 'the desire for motherhood is culturally induced, and the ability to mother is learned' (Oakley 1974). Girls are given dolls and doll's houses, while boys receive dinosaurs and racing cars. Interestingly, children as young as two often show preferences aligned with traditional gender roles.

These gender 'ideals' go much deeper than just what we choose to wear and play with – there is very much a 'script' regarding masculine and feminine qualities that many people follow, almost unconsciously. There is an unspoken narrative prevalent across many cultures that motherhood is the natural progression for women, and because it is seen as the norm it does not require additional training, intervention, or preparation. Instead, it is something that simply 'happens' to you, and once with child, the new mother is expected to flourish in her role due to the 'maternal instinct'.

Women worldwide are often expected to be nurturing and empathetic, with the aim of marrying and having children. In contrast, men are typically seen as dominant, independent, and focused on their careers, as the primary financial providers. Even in communities where these gender roles are reversed, the harsh reality is that these unspoken expectations can be deeply ingrained and difficult to change.

The elephant in the room – it takes a village

One of the most cherished memories from my youth was visiting Yala National Park in Sri Lanka. Home to 44 species of mammals and over 200 bird types, Yala is one of the world's most renowned wildlife sanctuaries, often called 'Leopard country' because it has one of the highest numbers of leopards globally. One animal we saw plenty of was my favourite, the Asian elephant. We watched five large elephants walking slowly, with a tiny elephant calf, just a few years old, weaving between them. I learned that elephant families keep their calves in the middle of the herd to protect them from falling behind or being attacked, adjusting their pace so the youngest can keep up.

Elephants have the longest pregnancy of any mammal, lasting about 22 months. This is not only due to their size but also their mental capacity. Elephants are regarded as some of the most intelligent animals on earth, comparable to chimpanzees and gorillas. At birth, they possess advanced neurodevelopment to learn from and imitate their elders for improved survival. Elephants also live in fully matriarchal societies, led by the oldest female, with family groups comprising daughters, sisters, and nieces. They can form deep emotional bonds, to such an extent that female relatives often 'babysit' and care for the offspring as if they were their own (Williams 2013).

What fascinates me is that when a baby is born to a mother, there are many similarities between elephants and humans. You may have heard the saying 'It takes a village to raise a child', which refers to the fact that raising a child is hard work, and most people would agree it requires support from others – a village – which could be the biological family (partner, parents, in-laws, aunts, siblings) or indeed the creation of your own 'village', such as neighbours, friends, childminders, nannies, or nursery support. Indra Nooyi, the former CEO of PepsiCo, reflects in her memoir on the early days of her career in senior management, navigating US business ideas with Indian home values, juggling the expectations of being a working mother. She describes this balance as the 'care ecosystem', where everyone rallied around the mother and the baby for them both to succeed in life (Nooyi 2021).

To summarise, in Chapter 4 I have introduced historical and cultural ideas of motherhood, and how we are programmed to feel a sense of love and responsibility for our children on a biological and social level. These high expectations placed on women provide fertile ground for the development of mental health issues in the perinatal period. In the next chapter, I will expose the myths of perfectionism and how this can influence both parenting and perinatal OCD.

CHAPTER 5

Motherhood, Parenting, and Perfectionism

For someone experiencing perinatal OCD, feelings of personal responsibility and the burden of perfectionism are often heightened. As we will examine in this section of the book, ideas of being a 'good enough mother' are frequently intertwined with fears of harm coming to their children. For any healthcare professional working in perinatal mental health, it is crucial to be aware of and curious about societal perceptions of women and parents, especially how these perceptions may be intensified when dealing with postnatal OCD and maternal perfectionism. In this chapter, I will explore perfectionism in detail, its relationship to maternal mental health, and how it may manifest from preconception to parenting, influencing behaviours and relationships.

THE GOOD ENOUGH MOTHER

As my maternity leave was ending, I was fortunate enough to spend an afternoon at the Hayward Gallery in London, exploring a vast yet intimate collection of key pieces of art by Louise Bourgeois. It was a lovely venture back into the real world, not only post-lockdown but also sans children, signalling the transitional end of my maternity leave and my return to clinical work.

The exhibition explored aspects of birth and mothering, focusing on both the child and the woman herself as she is 'birthed' into the role of motherhood. Bourgeois was able to articulate and express herself through beautifully intricate yet simple sculptures, paintings, and textiles. She experimented with various fabrics and objects, often contrasting one with another (delicate silk lingerie next to jagged wood, for example). I was in awe of her ability to manipulate several techniques, including weaving, embroidery, sculpture, quilting, printing, and painting. I have often felt that motherhood is juxtaposed in a similar way. Women may come with a textured past but often gloss over this in trying to define what they feel it must mean to be 'a good mother' – presenting a silky-smooth facade to the world.

One of her most renowned art installations is the Maman, a large, sprawling metallic spider sculpture made of steel, which earned her the fitting nickname, spider-woman. Louise describes the sculpture as 'an ode to [my] mother' and compares the spider to mothers, as they weave a web of family life and memories together while also being protective creatures that eat mosquitos, insects known to carry toxins and potentially cause harm. This mirrors the many mothers I meet who, within seconds of giving birth, undergo a complete overhaul of their priorities, roles, and responsibilities, where the 'maman' response becomes paramount. The matriarch emerges before our very eyes, and even when a child grows up, leaves home, and starts a family of their own, these somewhat primal instincts and the neurochemical rush of love and affection never truly fade, as being a mother remains central to her core identity.

Choosing a favourite piece from the exhibition is difficult, but if I had to pick one, it would be the sculpture of the Good Mother. It portrays a female figure kneeling, with her breasts connected to five spools of thread. The artwork evoked in me a powerful sense of sacrifice and selflessness, as the spools hang by a thread from her nipples while she displays a tired, forlorn expression. Of course, art invites multiple interpretations. A friend of mine saw it differently; where I perceived a burdened mother weighed down by her metaphorical children, he saw a mother as a master puppeteer, controlling her marionettes into chaos. Our contrasting yet equally valid perspectives likely reveal more about our backgrounds and views on motherhood – both real and imagined – than about the sculpture itself.

I have yet to meet a mother who hasn't experienced trying to be more than just 'good enough', often smiling through exhaustion. I also began to wonder what these spools represent in our busy modern lives. Louise Bourgeois created many works of art with themes centred around not only motherhood and parenting but also domesticity, childhood trauma, hidden emotions, mental health, sexuality, and the patriarchy. There are many things, places, and people, past and present, in our fantasy and reality, that we may hold on to, even if only by a thread. If you have worked with embroidery thread, you'll know that it may look delicate, but it is very strong and not easily broken. Being pulled in different directions, along with our efforts to meet expectations – both our own and those of other people – is enough to weigh anyone down. When working with women experiencing mental health issues, it is important to stay curious about the attachments in their lives – not just with their children but also with others, both in the present and the past.

What if good enough isn't enough?

Donald Winnicott famously wrote about the 'good enough mother', a mother with good intentions who can lay the foundations for a happy child (Winnicott 1967). However, how we mother and operate in the modern world has changed considerably since the 1960s. This shift has prompted me to reflect on Winnicott's work, and I have been preoccupied with the question: *What if good enough isn't enough?* Through a potent mix of capitalism and feminism in the second half of the 20th century, combined with the technological and digital advancements of the 21st century, some argue that women can truly 'have it all'. The bar has been raised, as have the expectations of women worldwide, who demand perfection from themselves and others. These types of mothers work hard and play hard, believing that if they can excel at work, in their physical appearance, or in their carefully curated lives reflected in aesthetically pleasing Instagram accounts, then why not apply this philosophy to their approach to mothering? Being 'good enough' implies average, mediocre, passable, ordinary. This implication conflicts with modern societal standards, which aim high and seek the extraordinary. In my clinical practice over the years, I've noticed that the common thread is that 'good enough' mothering doesn't inspire confidence or desirability; most mothers aspire to be *great*. Reflecting on the 'elephants in the room' – the insatiable hunger for perfectionism and control, especially during the perinatal period when so much remains unknown – can be deeply challenging for mothers and may sometimes precede mental health decline. With this in mind, in the following sections, we will explore the concept of perfection and how it is intricately woven into both motherhood and OCD.

WHAT IS PERFECTIONISM?

Perfectionism can be understood as the extent to which an individual strives to meet high, often unrealistic, standards. According to Hewitt and Flett (1991), perfectionism is a complex personality trait comprising three dimensions:

- self-oriented perfectionism (holding oneself to strict standards)
- other-oriented perfectionism (expecting perfection from others)
- socially oriented perfectionism (viewing others as demanding perfection, which can lead to a desire for approval and validation).

Although being a 'perfectionist' can bring many benefits and is often perceived positively, especially in areas such as competitive sports or career advancement, it is important to recognise that clinical perfectionism can sometimes cause stress and burnout and can negatively impact one's mental health and emotional wellbeing.

Perfectionism has been examined since the early 1950s, but research gained momentum in the 1970s when questions arose about whether perfectionism was simply a personality trait or potentially linked to psychopathology. Ortiz et al. (2022) found that high levels of perfectionism can increase the risk of mental health symptoms (such as depression and suicidal ideation) and are significantly comorbid with disorders like OCD and eating disorders. Specifically, these individuals may experience heightened anxiety about perfectionist actions, have difficulties in emotional regulation, pursue impulsive and often unachievable goals, and have a preoccupation with failure.

In the updated classification of the *International Classification of*

Diseases (ICD-11), perfectionism is not a standalone diagnosis but is recognised under the umbrella of obsessive-compulsive personality disorder, also known as anankastic personality disorder, which we will discuss more in Chapter 13. To qualify for a diagnosis, the perfectionism has to be of a severity and degree to cause enough distress to impact their overall quality of life. They navigate life as the captain of their well-organised ship, always in control and steadfastly following the carefully crafted path they have laid out. This approach tends to work well – that is, until they decide to start a family.

OCD and planning a pregnancy

Planning a pregnancy can be all-consuming, even for those without a diagnosis of OCD. Different influences such as travel and stress can affect whether ovulation is delayed or even happens (Bridges 2020). Women may engage in various behaviours and strategies when trying to conceive, including:

- ordering ovulation kits from the internet to test multiple times a day
- scheduling intercourse to align with predicted ovulation
- making changes to lifestyle and diet to improve chances of conceiving
- engaging beliefs and behaviours verging on superstitious (having sex in certain positions/times of day).

Waiting for a positive pregnancy test is an anxious time for many. Parents-to-be may fixate on every little sign, anxiously symptom-checking for indications of pregnancy before a test can confirm it. As discussed earlier in the book, this desire to start a family is largely accepted in our society. The pressure to conceive before the 'biological clock runs out' intensifies this preoccupation even more.

Many women who have been living with OCD and wish to start a family may find that their condition interferes with the process. This interference can occur in several ways, such as affecting their ability to be intimate (due to contamination fears) and leading to compulsive symptom checking while waiting to see if they have conceived. Once pregnant, there may be a marked deterioration in mood and mental state, with worsening pre-existing OCD symptoms or the emergence of a new cluster of symptoms, predominantly concerning the safety of the unborn baby. Feelings of anxiety and/or unwanted intrusive thoughts or images of horrific events happening to the baby *in utero* may arise. The fear of something happening to the baby *in utero* may be more prevalent in those who have previously experienced a traumatic event such as a miscarriage or stillbirth.

PERFECTIONISM AND PREGNANCY

Pregnancy can be a challenging time to navigate with perfectionistic ideals. Several aspects of the perinatal period (from conception, pregnancy, birth, and postnatal experience) cannot be controlled, and this lack of control is not only frustrating but potentially petrifying for those who struggle with perfectionism. Leaving something as important as becoming a mother to chance is too much for some. Consider the thousands of online forums dedicated to 'TTC' (trying to conceive) that offer endless advice on how, when, and even what position to 'DTD' (do the deed) to guarantee a positive pregnancy test in the first month. Ovulation calendars and prediction sticks bought in bulk online provide a sense of control in an uncontrollable situation, as studies show that even when all the timings line up perfectly and sex occurs at the right moment for the egg and sperm to meet, only 25% go on to become a viable embryo. The chances become even slimmer when you consider that only 25% of these 'successful' conceptions go on to become viable pregnancies, with one in five viable pregnancies not making it past the first trimester (Wilcox, Weinberg, & Baird 1995).

Each trimester presents its own unique uncertainties and risks to both the mother and the foetus. I have seen birth plans created with great care and good intentions (the ones that are eight pages printed double-sided and laminated) tossed aside in moments of chaos, and when sudden complications during labour demand emergency intervention. For those that struggle with perfectionism or the need to control outcomes, it is vital that this is identified early in the pregnancy, to allow for additional support from both the maternity and perinatal mental health team.

PERFECTIONISM IN THE POSTNATAL PERIOD

For some, the real challenge for perfectionists begins when the baby arrives and doesn't follow 'the rules'. As many of you know firsthand, babies have their own plans, especially during the first three months, often called the 'fourth trimester'. They have distinct sleep and wake cycles, feeding routines, and preferences. Some babies only sleep in their loved ones' arms, while others need loud white noise that can wake the neighbours.

Some perfectionists may find the nuances of their newborn easy to manage but then struggle to keep all the other plates spinning, such as household chores or the elusive 'work–life balance'. Perfectionism tendencies can come out of the woodwork during the postnatal period, and I often receive requests in clinic for permission about whether 'it's okay to leave the sink with dirty dishes' (it is). This reassurance is not just me providing practical solutions for women who come to me feeling desperately exhausted and burdened with maternal guilt, but rather a tested method of assessing how committed they are to their perfectionistic ways. For some, the simple advice and permission that it is okay to 'let go a bit' is all they need; they understand that this is temporary and lowering their high standards does not equate to a lowering of their worth as a woman or mother. However, for others, the advice is hard to accept. The feelings of control (or the distress of losing control) can be projected onto the prospective father, who may have a more relaxed, laissez-faire attitude towards parenting in comparison. There is, of course, another person to consider, and that is the child in the middle.

Perfectionistic parents often set unachievable standards for their children and see their successes or failures as a reflection of their parenting. They tend to reinforce what they value most – such as reaching developmental milestones, academic excellence, beauty standards, or talent in sports or music – and push these ideals onto the child. This can lead to the child struggling later in life under the pressure to meet these high expectations. Parents who have lived their lives striving for perfection may then find it difficult to accept an 'imperfect' child. In reality, there is a delicate balance between perfectionist ideals and the realities of adjusting to motherhood (Kawamoto & Furutani 2018; Lee, Schoppe-Sullivan, & Kamp Dush 2012).

Like in OCD, those with perfectionist personality traits may involve their partners and family in their perfectionist outlook. Unlike in OCD, perfectionists often have a strong belief that their worldview is 100% right, whereas a person with OCD may feel strongly that something is 'right' but be overwhelmed with doubt and seek reassurance more often than someone with perfectionism. This is where the lines between perfectionism and narcissism become blurred, as narcissists may take this unwavering conviction to the extreme of entitlement, believing it's 'my way or the highway', leaving little room for those who do not follow their rules. Although a fascinating topic, the concept of a narcissistic mother deserves another discussion, or even another book.

Perfectionists, by their nature, are often goal-focused and have a dichotomous 'all-or-nothing' mindset, favouring clear and objective 'pass-or-fail' situations and tasks. This can, of course, become problematic when it comes to parenting. Those with perfectionist tendencies may feel frustrated in relationships or parenting roles, as the other person in the dynamic (especially a baby) cannot be easily controlled or defined. Douglas and Michaels (2004) coined the term 'new momism', which describes a romanticised and demanding view of parenting, where standards are excessively high and nearly impossible to meet. This rising cultural phenomenon of 'parenting perfectionism' is reflected in social media, where maternal practices and patterns are shared online and subject to both praise and criticism from others, as discussed earlier in Part 1.

STRIVING TO BE THE PERFECT PARENT

Changes in socio-economic needs and cultural views on family influence these evolving trends. More people are choosing to delay parenthood until they complete higher education and secure stable jobs and finances. Furthermore, they are having fewer children than previous generations. Consequently, they have more time and resources to prepare for parenthood, which can create unrealistic expectations about parenting. Becoming a parent involves a significant societal responsibility, but it also offers wonderful rewards. Many people see it as one of the most fulfilling roles in life. In clinic, many women share their experiences, including those related to perinatal mental illness, and talk about how becoming a mother has been the most transformative and affirming journey for them – one they wouldn't trade for anything in the world.

As parental expectations continue to rise, investigating parental adjustment and perfectionism becomes increasingly important. Lee et al. (2012) collected longitudinal data from 182 couples and first-time parents in the US, assessing their parental adjustment during the third trimester and then at three, six, and nine months postnatally. They found that mothers experienced greater satisfaction and self-efficacy in their parenting roles compared to fathers. However, mothers also faced more societal perfectionism, being sensitive to the criticism and judgement of others regarding their mothering, whereas fathers displayed self-oriented perfectionism, being more motivated by personal achievement and success without the added pressure of comparison with other fathers. It is important to note that most study participants were married, white, heterosexual couples who were well-educated and financially stable. It would be valuable to re-examine these findings in different family types, such as single-parent households or those from diverse ethnic backgrounds or with socio-economic disadvantages.

Clark and Coker (2009) studied the links between maternal dysfunctional perfectionism and self-criticism in mothers and perfectionism and self-criticism in their teenage children. The study findings indicated a possible mechanism of perfectionism, noting that having high standards – and perceiving oneself to fall short of them – was often followed by a period of intense self-criticism and blame, which perpetuated a cycle of negative self-beliefs and feelings of maternal guilt and shame. Even if perfectionistic mothers meet the high standards they set for themselves, they may continue to set even higher goals, often just beyond their reach and therefore impossible to attain. This results in a recurring cycle of harsh self-criticism and feelings of low self-worth. Although the study did not find any statistically significant correlations, they did observe some links between perfectionism and self-criticism among mothers and daughters, compared to fathers and daughters.

Smith et al. (2017) also examined the relationships between over 200 mothers and daughters and the impact of maternal perfectionism. They found that women, in general, are more likely to experience societal perfectionism, which in turn leads to worse outcomes not only for the mothers but also for their daughters, resulting in increased stress and relationship breakdowns due to daughters feeling overly criticised and a deterioration of self-esteem. Feng, Zhang and Zhong (2021) believed that families exist within their own 'microsystem', where individuals are part of the family collective but are shaped by their upbringing, with parents playing a highly influential role in early childhood development. They delved deeper into parenting styles and found, in a study of 500 Chinese university students, that a positive parenting style and behaviours produce altruistic children, the development of positive peer relationships, and excellent social adaptability. Negative perfectionistic parenting styles, on the other hand, resulted in negative emotions in offspring and high levels of other-oriented perfectionism (in essence, wanting to meet the high expectations and wishes placed upon them by their parents). This study highlights the potential for cultural differences regarding parenting styles and levels of perfectionism around the world.

It is also worth noting that competing factors, beyond perfectionism, influence the high expectations of parents. For example, immigrant parents may place a strong emphasis on educational achievements for their children as a means of creating financial stability and/or cultural assimilation, believing that this will enhance the quality of life for future generations. I discuss parenting styles and the delicate balance of perinatal OCD and attachment styles further in Chapter 9.

PARENTING ONLINE: THE INFLUENCE OF SOCIAL MEDIA

An emerging and unexpected trend in how the influence of perfection affects our maternal mental health has been observed in our relationship with social media. The rise of online motherhood communities, parenting forums such as Mumsnet and Netmums, social media platforms like Facebook, Instagram, TikTok, and YouTube, and apps like Peanut, designed to foster social connections during the perinatal period, have created a microcosm of how we perceive maternal well-being and illness. Just a generation ago, making mum friends usually involved inviting someone over for a coffee or a playdate, or meeting at a local soft play or baby music class. Information sharing happened on a need-to-know basis, with only family members having a detailed understanding of your parenting styles and techniques. Now, this information is freely accessible to everyone. Even those who prefer to keep their family private can watch how others parent from the comfort of their own home.

While being able to observe, learn from, or critique others' parenting beliefs – such as their views on co-sleeping, gentle parenting, or weaning – comparisons can trigger strong feelings of maternal guilt, shame, and inadequacy, making one feel not like a 'good enough mum'. Shame has a social aspect, involving not only concern about how others might perceive you and your choices but also an internal expectation of what you believe others may think of you – regardless of whether they actually express any opinions. Alongside this, there is the rise of the mother-influencer, or 'mum-fluencer' – someone who identifies as a mother but also promotes themselves and their lifestyle, turning maternal identity into a 'brand' with a USP (unique selling point).

In clinical practice, we understand that not only is each child unique, but so is every mother. Although parenting fosters a sense of commonality among people, the depiction of motherhood online is often neither realistic nor attainable. Through the trials and tribulations of balancing motherhood and maternal identity, social media sites such as Facebook can be appealing as they offer not only a sense of community but also affirmation of strongly held beliefs about what it means to be a mum. Indeed, Schoppe-Sullivan et al. (2017) argue that new mothers use sites such as Facebook not only to seek support from others, but also as 'a platform to showcase to the world' that they are fulfilling their maternal roles as expected by society. Bartholomew et al. (2012) found that Facebook use increased when becoming a parent, despite the reduction in available time due to the increased tasks and responsibilities of new motherhood. The study also found that the integration of parenting on the internet has fostered a level of social connection, but evidence suggests that people are feeling lonelier and more isolated.

The internet, of course, is not all fake news. In 2016, I conducted a thematic discussion about perinatal OCD on internet chat forums. What transpired was astonishing. First, a large proportion of posts related to the inaccurate and lay understanding of being 'a bit OCD' (meaning someone who prefers things to be tidy, organised, and neat, or someone with a particular personality). Second, women were revealing symptoms and signs of their possible OCD during pregnancy and the postnatal period in a way never seen in clinical practice. Because of the anonymity of the posts, individuals were much more likely to discuss unwanted intrusive thoughts, including sexual or paedophilic fears, as well as concerns about inappropriate sexual thoughts and the fear of becoming aroused during breastfeeding, leading some to prefer bottle feeding. Some women even mentioned that they felt comfortable discussing these issues on forums like this with peer support, but would never do so with a health professional, due to fear and stigma surrounding maternal mental illness, and also a fear of being reported to social services or having their child taken away if they disclose this in person to their GP or health visitor.

In the final chapter of Part 2, I reflect on the duality of motherhood and OCD – the common challenges parents face with this condition (whether long-standing or new onset), but also the opportunities for us as health professionals to provide support during this challenging time.

CHAPTER 6

Motherhood and OCD

OCD AND CHALLENGES IN MOTHERHOOD

Most perinatal mental health services primarily support women during pregnancy and after childbirth, but there are also unspoken ways in which OCD can influence decisions about conception. This section explores how an OCD diagnosis might affect fertility or the choice to delay having children. It also considers how becoming a mother or experiencing a relapse of OCD symptoms can impact family dynamics and evoke feelings of loss. The chapter concludes by discussing a shared sense of protection, purpose, and empowerment in both motherhood and OCD, highlighting how understanding this balance can help us better support patients in distress.

Fertility

OCD and other mental health conditions can influence a person's journey to motherhood in various ways. Many women are aware of their 'biological clock' and the reality of declining fertility, and several countries are now facing a potential population crisis due to low birth rates (Kim & Lee 2020). Men, however, do not seem to face the same time constraints regarding fertility, with many fathering children well into their 50s, 60s, and even 70s, while women over 37 in maternity services are labelled as having 'geriatric' pregnancies.

Women may feel anxious about conceiving or delay having children due to unresolved mental health issues, some of which could be specific to OCD. This, along with the known prevalence of latent OCD diagnoses in the general population and the tendency of many women to pursue further education and career development instead of the traditional idea of 'settling down', puts young women in a difficult position.

In clinical practice, this could mean a couple with differing views and ideas about parenthood. It is not uncommon for one partner to be keener on having a baby than the other, or for one to feel pressured to have a baby. Fertility struggles can significantly affect not only the couple's relationship but also their individual mental health, and there is evidence to suggest an increased risk of psychological distress and anxiety-related disorders among those with assisted pregnancies (Sharma & Shrivastava 2022).

Those experiencing OCD may face additional and unique challenges on top of the already stressful issue of trying to conceive. We know that for many people with OCD, they may conceal their symptoms or go without a formal diagnosis for many years; thus, the condition may remain undetected, undiagnosed, and untreated even before conception. The process of fertility treatments may also trigger anxiety, obsessive thoughts, and compulsive behaviours, through checking for ovulation and pregnancy symptoms or increased reassurance-seeking. I explore this further in Chapter 8.

Delaying conception

Putting off having children may also be part of OCD presentation and symptomatology – where avoidance plays a significant role in the condition (due to fear of harm coming to their children, or ego-dystonic thoughts of a sexual nature, worried that having a child may confirm their intrusive and disturbing worries of being a paedophile, for example, thus logically feeling it is better not to be near children at all). Additionally, many women may delay childbirth due to fears that their children might inherit their OCD, concerns that their mental health could deteriorate during the perinatal period, or apprehensions about taking medication during pregnancy and breastfeeding.

Family dynamics

Family involvement can be a double-edged sword. Even without pre-existing mental health issues, tensions may emerge between generations due to differences in parenting styles and family dynamics. In the context of a new or existing OCD diagnosis, many families may have already adopted relational patterns and routines to manage OCD symptoms for years, making these behaviours so familiar that they go unquestioned. There may be unspoken tensions or pressure to continue following certain rules and rituals during the perinatal period, such as reassurance-seeking, excessive checking, or washing rituals, which may also extend to caring for the baby.

OCD symptoms in the mother may worsen if family members who previously were willing to participate in the compulsive behaviours decide they no longer want to support this, set boundaries on involvement, or choose to do things differently in a way that doesn't align with the mother's OCD when caring for the newborn. For some women, the transition into motherhood is filled with anxiety. I have lost count of how many women have visited my clinic crying about their relationships with their mothers (and mothers-in-law) – the common theme being their feelings of failing to meet the expectations of what they believe a mother should be. It can be quite difficult to live in the shadow of an experienced mother (especially when you are literally under the same roof), made harder by a lack of confidence in their own parenting abilities, especially if it is their first time. I discuss the role of family in therapeutic recovery more in Chapter 16.

I'm turning into my mother

'Oh my God. I'm turning into my mother!' I remember a patient saying to me, half laughing and half wincing as she tried to soothe her teething child in an outpatient clinic. Although this exclamation is often uttered in jest, the truth behind this realisation can be a shock to the new mother, who has vowed in her own mind, even before conception, that she will be 'nothing like her'. It often begins with just a word or a passing phrase she recalls her mother saying to her when she was a child, which she unconsciously repeats to her own child, triggering the memory.

Even in the closest maternal relationships, a new pregnancy signifies a rebirth; it is an opportunity to reimagine a new chapter, a fresh start, a new life, and, importantly, a chance for the daughter to branch out and become a mother herself with her own ideas and beliefs. This can, however, be challenging for a first-time mother, as the role is entirely new, and she is essentially learning on the job. Who else can she learn from but the example set by her primary caregiver (who, in most cases but not all, is the biological mother)? Becoming a mother is akin to putting on ice skates and stepping onto a frozen lake, uncertain of how thick the ice is beneath, in constant fear it may crack, and that it could subside at any moment. Part of our role as health professionals is to instil confidence in the uncertain mother, to tune in to her own understanding of her child, and to nurture her self-belief in her abilities, especially if she feels overly critiqued and judged by others (which may exist within or outside mental illness).

LOSSES IN MOTHERHOOD

Motherhood brings great joy and is seen as a blessing by many. Even those who experience loss often find ways to balance this with their positive gains. We must also acknowledge that some women are navigating their roles as mothers during times of loss, even when these moments are meant to be the happiest moments of their lives. This loss might involve their own parent, a significant relationship, or a previous child through miscarriage, stillbirth, or neonatal death. Sadly, many in this latter group often fall through the gaps of perinatal mental health services.

It is important not to over-pathologise these women by confusing grief with a mental illness, and to recognise that the pain and suffering may require specialised care for those who might be vulnerable to developing psychological difficulties in the future if their needs are ignored. Those who have lost their mothers (through death or distance) or who have an estranged relationship with them may feel as if they have been left to navigate this new world alone, as if they are driving through heavy fog with the lights set to full beam yet unable to see the road ahead.

As a clinician caring for such women, you may find yourself taking up a surrogate maternal role; someone that will listen, provide reassurance, offer hope during the tough times, and celebrate the milestones. Do not underestimate your importance to these women at such a pivotal time in their lives, as they will look back and be thankful for all that you did to support them during a huge transition in their lives. It is not uncommon for children centres and primary care, perinatal mental health, maternity, and health visiting services to become that 'village' for women and their children in the early years. This is particularly true for women who are isolated for one or more of several reasons, including migrant women, victims of domestic violence and abuse, and those who are mothering alone even whilst in relationships with their partner working long hours or away from home. Of course, women with perinatal OCD may also be isolated and vulnerable for additional reasons, such as feeling anxious and avoidant of leaving the house due to obsessional fears (of contamination/safety of the baby, etc.).

'Just Mummy' – the loss of self

There is, of course, a more subtle form of loss that accompanies motherhood: the loss of a previous life and the person we used to know 'pre-kids'. I have often heard women complain that, although they love their children dearly, they frankly feel irritated at being seen as 'just Mummy'. Health services also reinforce this single identity by often calling women 'Mum' instead of their first name during consultations. What is usually a term of endearment and creates a sense of community can also feel suffocating, eroding the life we once had and slowly diminishing our sense of self. Combined with physical changes of motherhood – including stress incontinence, haemorrhoids, leaking nipples, breast changes, hair loss, pain during sex, reduced libido, caesarean section scars, and softer belly – it is not surprising that one might feel alien to her past self. These changes, coupled with the mental load of parenting and managing a household, can be overwhelming (Sicard et al. 2021).

The loss of self, both emotionally and physically, is coupled with another strange sense of loss of personal space. As a mother of two beautiful young girls, I have not only been a mother but a provider of nourishment, a climbing frame, a punching bag, a cuddle giver, a singer and rocker to sleep. I have been pinched, poked, prodded, pushed, pulled, and what some describe as being 'touched out'. Body autonomy is an unusual but important reflection here. A mother who has fears about touch and contamination might prefer to avoid such situations, which can be difficult in a caring role for children.

There is also a loss of personal space within the healthcare system – women will have the most encounters with health professionals during the perinatal period compared to the rest of their lives. Those experiencing OCD (and equally those who aren't) may feel uncomfortable with frequent touch and examinations by health professionals, especially during intimate examinations that are essential during labour. Women who have experienced sexual assault and/or abuse may have increased sensitivity to this, and we will discuss this later in the book in relation to the parallels between OCD and trauma.

Although the joy of being a mother is irreplaceable, some women may feel a sense of loss for the life they might have had if they were not tied to the daily grind and responsibilities of parenting. Missed career opportunities, travel, or even just the idea of an entirely different lifestyle without children can weigh on mothers, especially those struggling during the baby phase of motherhood where the days are long but the years feel short. It is not only a loss of personal identity but also a loss of vocation, as those who have spent years trying to establish a career or business path may find a lengthy maternity leave a daunting prospect or face job uncertainty.[1] For those with perinatal OCD, the structure of work may provide containment or distraction from their illness or be embedded in their daily compulsive rituals. For these women, maternity leave, or becoming a 'stay-at-home mum', can be especially stressful.

OCD AND MOTHERHOOD: THE THREE PS

Based on my research into the maternal experience and my clinical practice with thousands of women and mothers over the years, I have identified three overlapping themes shared in OCD and motherhood. When these themes are balanced, they lead to a positive and fulfilling mothering experience; when they are imbalanced, they can

1 Pregnant Then Screwed is a charity campaigning for change in this area: https://pregnantthenscrewed.com

cause disharmony and challenges. These perceptions often develop as the parent–infant relationship evolves, from nurturing a newborn to managing life after the 'empty nest'. I believe these themes are universal, regardless of ethnicity, sexual orientation, age, or education level, connecting mothers from all backgrounds through a shared significant experience. Figure 6.1 illustrates three major themes that I believe unify mothers worldwide, and these concepts may also shed light on our understanding of perinatal OCD.

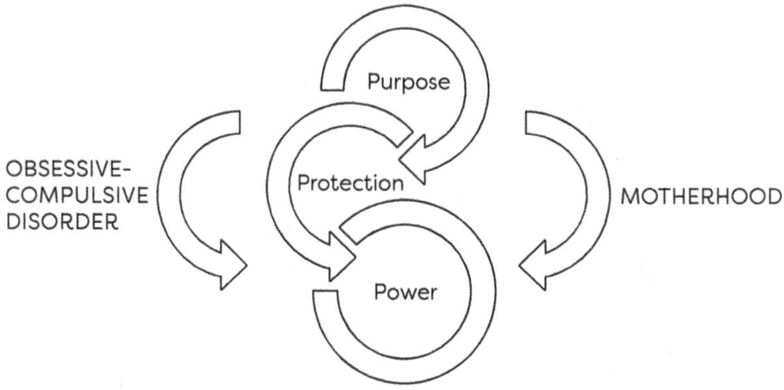

Figure 6.1 Parallels of OCD and motherhood

Sense of purpose

Despite the circumstances surrounding conception or birth, the very act of bringing life into the world can offer a sense of purpose as a new role of 'mother' is formed, and this 'job', as it were, is lifelong. For some, this role becomes all-encompassing, especially in those early years when the baby is 100% dependent on its caregiver. Of course, it can also go the other way; those who find the imposed title that comes with the territory of mothering difficult may shy away from the role and its responsibilities. This can manifest in many ways, but, when extreme, it can leave children vulnerable and at risk of neglect (unless another adult can step in as a primary caregiver).

OCD can truly feel all-encompassing because it's both obsessive and compulsive by its very nature. Some individuals have been living with the condition since childhood, which makes it hard to imagine life without it. It often becomes a part of who they are, and friends and family might find themselves 'walking on eggshells' to stay within what's acceptable or offering repeated reassurance. While one might be cautious to say that OCD gives a kind of 'purpose' to their lives – meaning a sense of value and significance – it can, in some ways, genuinely provide a sense of purpose, in the truest sense of the word.

In OCD, beliefs, behaviours, and actions are all centred around obsessional fears and compulsive acts, which help make sense of the irrational fears we experience inside. Without pairing these obsessions with compulsions, it's easy to get stuck on tangible fears that can increase anxiety and discomfort, leaving us feeling confused and unsettled instead of clear and purposeful. On a journey of recovery and self-discovery – whether you're undergoing OCD treatment or a mother reclaiming your independence after those tough early years – it's important to recognise the potential emptiness that the condition or children might leave behind. That's why it's so important to be gentle with yourself during this time, to find a new balance of purpose, and to rediscover who you are beyond any labels of OCD or motherhood.

Sense of protection

Like purpose, both motherhood and OCD share a commonality of protection. Defence mechanisms are natural in the wild – there is the example of female bears and their cubs, often colloquially referred to as the 'Mama Bear' instinct. Bear cubs, like babies, are especially vulnerable to dangers and threats from the outside world during their first year of life. A study of brown bears in Alaska found female bears to exhibit a wide range of responses in protecting their young – not only by being aggressive on the attack but also by defending their cubs and choosing to avoid confrontation when necessary (Berg 2020). This can be likened to learned and adapted behaviours in OCD – the compulsive response to fear can be multifaceted, including anger, repetitiveness, and avoidance of triggering situations.

Protection, however, is a double-edged sword – overprotection of children can be harmful and limiting, while too little protection may indicate concern and even border on child neglect. In my perinatal clinic, I often say that a little anxiety is essential for a new mother – part of being a responsible caregiver involves being aware of the dangers and risks around the child; parents of young children instinctively move a cup of hot tea away from the edge of the table, just in case of spillage. If there was no anxiety at all, I would be more worried, as this could leave the child vulnerable to potential harm, whether from child abuse or neglect.

Sense of power

Having a sense of power or control is a key theme that resonates deeply with both individuals dealing with OCD and new parents. During a child's first year, the parent truly becomes their child's world – caring for all their needs, from bathing to feeding, playing, and comforting. Humans are quite special in this way – though newborns can hear, see, taste, and smell from birth, they rely entirely on their parents for both practical care and emotional support. As Peter Parker (also known as Spiderman) was famously told by his uncle, 'With great power comes great responsibility.'

In OCD, many of the obsessional thoughts and compulsive rituals serve as ways to ease anxiety. People with OCD often try to control their environment – like deep cleaning the entire house or repeatedly asking family members to wash their hands – to feel more in control and calmer inside. Family members and partners often go along with these behaviours to maintain harmony and avoid upsetting the person with OCD, which can make them feel like they are taking the lead in the relationship dynamics.

The risk of this power imbalance becomes especially concerning when it affects the vulnerable newborn. In clinical practice, it's quite rare for mothers to impose their OCD fears directly onto their babies, such as insisting on frequent washing or using disinfectants on the baby. Instead, they often prefer to avoid certain situations or take responsibility for cleaning themselves to protect their little ones as much as possible. In most of my cases with mothers going through perinatal OCD, their caring and attentive approach to their babies has been inspiring, with the main goal being to minimise harm rather than add to it. Of course, clinicians need to stay aware of the safeguarding risks, which we'll delve into later in this book.

With all of this in mind, it is no surprise that motherhood can feel like a battlefield, and experiencing OCD during this vulnerable time has you surrounded and under attack. The ideas and expectations of motherhood, coupled with one's own strict criteria and standards as part of the OCD illness, can be difficult to balance, with many women describing feeling exhausted and drained trying to keep up with not just being a mother but the silent demands the illness places upon them. Particularly in those early sleep-deprived years, when the years feel short, but the days are long, the blurred lines between overwhelm and becoming unwell are too apparent. With the complexities that women face during the perinatal years, one common thread I have encountered through my clinical practice is that mothers who not only survive mental illness in the perinatal period but continue to thrive in the years that follow are those who taken the time to reflect on their own relationship with themselves and others, in particular their understanding of the concept of motherhood and family. The prevailing theme that unifies their recovery through even the darkest of moments is the allowing of emotional space to create their own meaning of motherhood, free of restraint from the ideas, concerns, and expectations of others, which, of course, is easier said than done. In Part 3, we explore deeper into the intertwined histories of OCD and women's mental illness that have shaped our modern-day appreciation of perinatal OCD.

PART 3

UNDERSTANDING PERINATAL OCD

In Part 3, I examine perinatal OCD from a broad and enriching perspective that includes historical, neuroscientific, and psychoanalytical insights. While these aspects may initially seem disconnected, they beautifully underpin society's perception of mental health needs during the perinatal period, helping us deepen our understanding of the condition. I present an overview spanning approximately 2000 years, during which the conceptions of OCD and perinatal mental health have developed in parallel, yet intriguingly share similar characteristics. Recognising the challenges women have faced throughout history in the treatment of mental illness allows us to better understand the stigmas and stereotypes they still confront today, often labelled as 'hysterical' or 'neurotic'. The neurobiological and psychological factors influencing perinatal OCD also inform common questions put to health professionals in clinical practice. Many parents may worry about potentially passing on their OCD to their children – whether through inherited genetics or parenting behaviours.

CHAPTER 7

History of Perinatal OCD

OCD and mental illness in motherhood are intricately linked, woven together throughout history with parallel themes. It is essential to acknowledge that much of the historical literature on OCD and mental illness during the perinatal period was written by men of European Caucasian descent in a time of prevailing Christian orthodox thinking. Thus, one must be mindful that the understanding of the illness is viewed through the eyes and observations of this somewhat narrow lens. It is only in the 20th century, through the works of Freud and the 'mothers of psychoanalysis' (see the box below), that women and children were not only seen but also heard. These works allowed us to delve deeper into the realm of mother and baby attachment during the perinatal period and its impact on mental illness.

HYSTERIA: A WOMAN'S DISEASE

The term 'hysteria' was first used by Hippocrates in the 5th century BCE. It originates from the Greek word *hysterikos* (suffering of the womb) and has long served as the encompassing phrase for anxiety spectrum disorders and trauma, which were historically deemed a 'woman's disease'. Not only did the word's meaning associate and restrict the illness to women, but it also confined it to the female reproductive organs, necessitating various manipulations for the anxiety to be 'removed' (Cleghorn 2021).

Perinatal mental illness and OCD have a common thread of religious and moral preoccupation. Women were both shamed and blamed for their mental illness. In the 12th century, it was believed that women were overly pious, which led to increased levels of anxiety and dissatisfaction. Indulging in the freedoms of the flesh and pleasing their male partners was thought to be the remedy, leading to greater satisfaction and reduced levels of stress. By the 1300s, the moral compass had swung in the opposite direction. Women's promiscuity was believed to be the root cause of their mental anguish, as well as the downfall of their partners (Tasca et al. 2012). Chastity became the treatment of choice for deranged and delinquent women, a reflection of the hyper-religious era.

Religion significantly influenced the origins of OCD. Religious texts from the 1400s describe intense anxiety about sin and obsessional religious themes. One example involves a German theologian who wrote about a Catholic nun convinced that her confessions were 'not sufficient'. Tragically, she died from excessive fasting to atone for her sins (OCD-UK 2025c). These traits remain common in OCD symptoms today. To combat religious ruminations, ritualistic behaviours like praying multiple times a day and cleansing are not uncommon. I discuss the intricate relationship between OCD and religious practices further in Chapter 10.

OBSESSION, OPPRESSION, OR POSSESSION?

During the Middle Ages, obsession became synonymous with hostile possession by evil spirits. Women struggling with mental health issues, or those trying to nurse those affected, were considered to be witches. Death by public hanging became the price they paid for their crimes. Sadly, historical accounts confirm that women who exhibited symptoms of mental illness continued to be mistreated and institutionalised well into the 20th century. As scientific theory became more prominent, evidence-based practice trumped the religious doctrines of previous generations.

In 1895, Sigmund Freud described *Zwangneurose*, translated as 'compulsion neurosis', as 'the instant impulse to behave in a certain way'. The Rat Man case study, in which Freud outlined the psychoanalytical treatment of a 29-year-old man who developed specific impulses against aggressive and sexual obsessions, is widely considered the original study of an OCD illness. It draws upon Freud's theories of mental structure and our mostly unconscious psychological defence mechanisms. This involves the conflict between the id (our inner unconscious desires, which may be aggressive or sexual by nature) and the ego, leading to behaviours considered 'embarrassing' or socially unacceptable (Freud 1909). European scholars continued to argue that OCD was characterised by the presence of intrusive ideas or images in the mind, and, importantly, against a person's will (Oberbeck, Stengler, & Steinberg 2013). Although medications became available (such as lithium, first prescribed for bipolar disorder in 1948), psychotherapy was the preferred treatment of choice. These theories remained well accepted until the 1960s. From that point, modern understandings of psychological theory and practice, such as cognitive behavioural therapy, took centre stage in our theoretical understanding of OCD (Brune 2006; Moritz et al. 2011).

Mothers of Psychoanalysis

Freud did not specifically treat perinatal mental health conditions. He did however develop a specific interest in hysteria, co-authoring *Studies on Hysteria* with the physician Josef Breuer in 1895 and later publishing the paper 'Female sexuality', written after his mother's death. He and his contemporaries believed that neuroses and hysteria were predominantly an emotional rather than medical issue, rooted in repressed trauma and sexual conflict (Bogousslavsky & Dieguez 2014). Labelling someone as 'hysterical' or 'neurotic' almost always related to a woman (Schafer 1974). Freud's theories have since been discredited; however, the symbolism of the 'hysterical woman' remains in contemporary culture.

The emergence of a new wave of female psychotherapists (aptly referred to as the mothers of psychoanalysis) ran with Freud's ideology but also embraced concepts around motherhood, sexuality, and the importance of mother–baby attachment and the family unit (Sayers 1993). Helene Deutsch, Karen Horney, Anna Freud, and Melanie Klein, all of whom were students of Freud, brought a matriarchal spin and displayed the courage to challenge and critique the paternalistic approach of psychoanalysis that they had been taught. Their contributions coincided with the rise of third-wave feminism and a societal shift towards greater autonomy for women, such as the wider availability of contraception to all women in the 1960s. These changes provided agency for young women to make choices about their body and reproductive life in a way that was never an option to them before (Jayarajah & Seneviratne 2016).

FRENCH CONTRIBUTIONS

Nineteenth-century Paris became the epicentre of significant advancements in the diagnosis of OCD, with French psychiatrist Jean Esquirol first describing it as a form of monomania, or partial insanity, in his 1838 psychiatric textbook. Further understanding was provided by notable French psychiatrists, including Henri Dagonet, Théodule-Armand Ribot, Charles Féré, Frédéric Paulhain, and Pierre Janet. Between the 1830s and early 1900s, French psychiatrists, psychologists, and philosophers generally concurred that OCD was an emotional disorder characterised by a pathological condition related to the dysregulation of the autonomic nervous system. Philosophers debated whether OCD was a disease of volition or impulse. The discussion surrounding the condition not only reflects the confusion and lack of clarity of the time but also highlights how OCD, much like its presentation today, is often misunderstood and 'pigeonholed' into pre-existing mental health conditions rather than treated (Berrios 1989).

Around the same time, the French were also leading the way in the understanding of perinatal mental illness. In 1858, Louis-Victor Marcé published the seminal *Treatise on Insanity in Pregnant, Postpartum, and Lactating Women*. This extensive collection of literature surveyed existing knowledge of psychiatric disorders that affect women during and after pregnancy. This work included 79 case studies featuring clinical presentations of severe postnatal depression and psychosis, paving the way for the establishment of perinatal mental health services and recognising that women present differently and are at a higher risk during the perinatal period. Although Marcé did not explicitly discuss cases of maternal OCD, he acknowledged broader categories of melancholia, mania, and monomania, as well as the crucial role pregnancy can play in increasing vulnerability to mental health issues. Marcé is regarded as the 'father of perinatal mental illness'. His name adorns the esteemed Marcé Society, the international centre for research and education in perinatal mental illness (Trede et al. 2009).

KEEP CALM AND CARRY ON: THE ADVANCEMENT OF PERINATAL PSYCHIATRY IN BRITAIN

In London during the 1950s and 1960s, child psychiatrist Dr John Bowlby became widely recognised as the 'father of attachment theory' through his pioneering work. In 1951, Bowlby wrote *Maternal Care and Mental Health* for the World Health Organization. This report was based on clinical findings concerning the effects of World War II on mothers and children, particularly the impact of the Blitz in London. These bombings created a unique situation of child separation from their mothers as they were evacuated from London, referred to as the 'Pied Piper Project' (Bowlby 1951). Although Bowlby faced some criticism for the lack of empirical evidence and statistical data, his report was extremely influential and significant for the era. It was one of the first pieces of evidence that led the government to reconsider its approach to maternal mental health and to understand that a mother and infant should not be separated during times of ill health and distress. Bowlby's work demonstrated immediate and long-term effects on a child's social, emotional, and cognitive development (Bretherton 1992).

Understanding the historical evolution of obsessive-compulsive disorder – from its early conceptualisations as religious or moral failings to its classification as a distinct psychiatric condition – provides essential context for the advances of modern neuroscience. The shift from spiritual interpretations to psychological and biological models reflects broader changes in society's views regarding both women and mental illness over the centuries. Today, cutting-edge neuroimaging, genetics, and cognitive neuroscience enable us to explore the underlying circuitry of OCD, which will be examined in the next chapter. This bridge between historical perspectives and contemporary science not only deepens our understanding of OCD's mechanisms but also affirms the importance of integrating clinical insight with biological advancements to inform more effective, personalised treatments.

CHAPTER 8

Understanding the Neuroscience of Perinatal OCD

OCD is a complex condition with various schools of thought regarding its causal origins, including psychological, biological, and cognitive factors. This chapter reviews the neuroscience of perinatal OCD, specifically neurobiology, genetics, and environmental factors, and the impact of female hormones.

WHAT NEUROBIOLOGY REVEALS

Currently, there are no published clinical or research studies specifically looking at the neurobiology or neuroanatomy of OCD presenting in pregnant women or mothers. The neurobiological basis of perinatal OCD remains a mystery. Our understanding of it relies on 'borrowing' from studies of mostly men presenting with OCD, coupled with our somewhat primitive understanding of the biology of maternal bonding and attachment.

The gender gap in research may be, in part, due to ethical and safety considerations concerning pregnant women participating in studies (such as the use of fMRI during pregnancy). However, there is scope for further studies in this under-researched area to deepen our understanding of whether the neurobiological or genetic origins of OCD in women or perinatal OCD differ from those seen in men and/or the non-perinatal population (Lochner & Stein 2011; Mattina & Steiner 2016). Thanks to the confirmation of several neuroscientific studies in the general population, we can now safely assume that OCD is directly related to brain circuitry, specifically the connection between the orbitofrontal area and the basal ganglia. This is further evidenced by the emergence of OCD symptoms in other neurological disorders affecting the basal ganglia, such as Tourette syndrome and Huntington's disease. Additional evidence has come from both new-onset OCD symptoms in those with focal brain injury (particularly affecting the frontal-subcortical area) and advancements in neuroimaging research, which allow us to visualise key areas of brain activity that 'light up' when OCD is present (Nakao, Okada, & Kanba 2014).

'You've got mail': OCD and the brain

The prefrontal area of the brain (specifically, the oribitofrontal cortex) sits above and behind the eyes. It is believed to be responsible for decision-making and impulse control, as well as matters of emotional and social concerns, such as guilt, acting inappropriately, and personal hygiene. The basal ganglia is a collection of connected structures in the mid-brain. These govern our motor control (movements) as well as our emotions, learning, and addictive behaviours.

These two areas are in constant communication. Every second of every day, the basal ganglia receives, organises, and filters a constant stream of thought sent from the prefrontal cortex. Like the ultimate productivity system, the basal ganglia receives a 'brain dump' to-do list of information, identifies urgent and non-urgent tasks and prioritises urgent tasks for immediate action. In OCD, however, the 'inbox' gets filled up so fast with messages that the brain is unable to keep up and process what needs a reply or what can go in the trash bin as spam. When every message is seen as important and urgent, the brain's circuits can become overwhelmed, giving rise to obsessional beliefs and compulsive actions.

A high-level explanation of the neurobiological theory of OCD suggests that overactivity in the orbitofrontal area gives rise to a preoccupation with obsessional thoughts and images. When faced with something one perceives as a danger or threat, the orbitofrontal cortex sends messages to the basal ganglia. This, in turn, activates the direct (excitatory) and indirect (inhibitory) circuits within the basal ganglia (Mataix-Cols & van den Heuvel 2012).

In a non-OCD brain, the danger signals are recognised and alleviated by the direct pathway. Meanwhile, the indirect pathway stops further signals (and thus actions) firing in a feedback-loop mechanism. In the OCD brain, however, the direct pathway is 'over-excited' and overrides the delicate balance provided by the indirect feedback loop. This translates, clinically, into an overvaluation/obsessional rumination about a particular worry, threat, or fear, which is then put on repeat in the brain without a clear 'off-switch'.

For example, someone may be worried about a possible terrorist threat while at their workplace. In a person with a non-OCD brain, they might have a fleeting thought or an unwanted distressing image in their mind. They are, however, quickly (and often subconsciously) able to reassure themselves through a swift mental calculation of probability and risk (the situation around them is calm, there has never been a terrorist threat in their workplace, no warnings have been issued, and the building is in an area that is not considered high risk or threatened by terrorism). The indirect pathway ensures that the thought remains 'one-off' and insignificant, allowing the individual to go about their day, enjoy their work, and return home safely without delays.

In OCD, however, this feedback mechanism is faulty. The person becomes overwhelmed by intense thoughts of worry and fear about a terrorist attack occurring at their workplace, which may also include distressing visual images of burning buildings or maimed bodies. These heightened danger signals are picked up by the basal ganglia, which set in motion behaviours to reduce the distress. However, as the direct pathway is so prominent, it dominates the indirect pathway that would have communicated to the orbitofrontal cortex to stop signalling danger and/or to indicate that the person is indeed safe. Thus, the firing of the unfiltered perceived threat continues on repeat, giving rise to frequent, unwanted, distressing thoughts and images that are obsessional in nature. These are accompanied by a host of protective and often elaborate behaviours or rituals one must perform to neutralise the danger. Such behaviours may include repeating certain phrases or a sequence of numbers that the person believes will guarantee safety or tapping the desk and the computer in a specific pattern to create a sense of security. Other compulsive symptoms include reassurance-seeking behaviours (asking co-workers repeatedly if there is any security threat, checking the fire alarms or CCTV) or indeed the most obvious and over-looked behaviour – avoidance (not going to work at all, thus not placing oneself in danger in the first place).

These thoughts can be really tough for someone to handle, and the compulsive behaviours that come up in an attempt to manage them can sometimes spiral out of control. When these issues are not addressed, they might interfere not just with daily work, but also with relationships with colleagues, and could ultimately put their job at risk. Imagine a fear or worry emerging in a mother, whether she has new-onset or pre-existing OCD. It's understandable to wonder whether the significant biological and hormonal changes during pregnancy and the postpartum period could explain why her protective instinct might go into overdrive. We often hear that being overprotective and deeply caring for a newborn is seen as normal behaviour for mothers, and some even rationalise being 'obsessed' with their baby. But what if this care opens floodgates of worry that feel impossible to shut off? We can start by examining the neuro-biology of perinatal mental health disorders and recent evidence regarding the genetic, environmental, and hormonal influences on both the mother and developing foetus.

OCD AND GENETICS

The genetic basis of OCD and related health conditions has experienced a resurgence over the last 20 years, driven by the completion of the human genome sequence. This international collaborative research programme began in 1990 and concluded in 2003. For the first time in history, researchers mapped the complete genetic blue-print for humankind. This ignited a new generation of deeper exploration into genetics and its impact on our health.

As with other areas of neuroscientific research, our understanding of OCD, particularly perinatal OCD, is limited and under-studied. Despite these limitations, it is important for the genetic aspect of OCD to be addressed in this book. Not only is OCD and genetics a fascinating, emerging field of evidence-based research, but the concept of genetic heritability frequently arises in clinical settings for pregnant individuals who are concerned about the possibility of passing down their mental illness to their children. Below, I summarise the latest developments in genetic research concerning OCD, along with the environmental factors that can influence the development of OCD in children (Grisham, Anderson, & Sachdev 2008).

Keeping it in the family: Twin/family studies

The question of whether OCD is a familial condition that can be passed down through generations via genetic means has been asked for nearly a century, with the first studies published in the 1930s. Early genetic research of twin studies and family lineage studies show some evidence of OCD running in families (e.g. Krebs et al. 2015; van Grootheest et al. 2005); however, the studies are small and use differing methodologies, making it hard to generalise the findings. In twin studies we see a 50% increased risk of OCD in identical twins, compared with non-identical twins (Samuels 2009). This finding begs the question of whether environmental factors are at play (more on this later). Other studies show 'family clusters' of OCD of up to four affected generations. However, it is widely agreed that cases such as this are the exception to the rule (Mahjani et al. 2021; Mataix-Cols et al. 2013). OCD often presents as sporadic, with no one else in the family displaying symptoms. One must also be mindful that we pass much more than genes from parent to child, and from generation to generation: familial views, cultural beliefs, emotional connections, and communication styles.

Molecular genetics and polymorphisms

Further studies have focused on whether conditions such as OCD are linked to a particular aspect of the genetic code. Some have explicitly attempted to find a 'risk' gene located in a specific area of the chromosome, or whether changes in the DNA sequence could impact the clinical manifestation of obsessive and compulsive symptoms. Most studies have been inconclusive and unable to pinpoint a specific gene that is responsible for the condition (Bloch et al. 2008; Stewart et al. 2013).

New research in molecular genetics has focused on 'candidate' genes that code for information processing via neurochemical pathways in the brain. Specifically, several genes that influence the serotonergic, dopaminergic, and glutamatergic pathways in the brain's circuitry have been linked to OCD expression (Purty et al. 2019, Sinopoli et al. 2017). This has relevance not only for strengthening the neurobiological hypothesis of OCD but also for pharmacological treatment options. An example of this is the early research and consideration of glutaminergic drugs like memantine for treatment of OCD (Ferguson et al. 2023; Grados et al. 2013; Maiti et al. 2023).

However, OCD is more than just a mere short-circuit of the brain. Seeking the golden ticket is akin to searching for a tiny needle in a barn full of haystacks. Our understanding of genes has evolved over time. We now appreciate that there are not only gene–environment interactions but also gene–gene interactions. Functional polymorphism suggests that the scope of genetic influence is vast and not solely biological in nature. Genes can influence both physical and personal characteristics, such as cognitive processing patterns and traits associated with perfectionism, which may make a person more susceptible to developing OCD. The more we explore OCD, the more we understand that the condition itself comprises several subthemes and niche presentations. OCD may be coded differently for men and women, across different ethnicities, and among specific populations such as pregnant and postnatal women, and this may have clinical implications such as response to therapy (Behesti et al. 2023; Dondu, Caliskan, & Orenay-Boyacioglu 2022; Mak, Streiner, & Steiner 2015).

Back to the future: The discovery of GWAs

The most promising research to date on a genetic theory of OCD involves the relatively recent discovery of genome-wide associations (GWAS, affectionately referred to and pronounced as 'gee-waahs' by researchers in the field). It is a research method where geneticists can scan the entire genome of a targeted population (such as those with OCD) to identify common genetic markers. Still in its infancy, this research explores whether certain conditions are associated with specific areas of the genetic map.

To date, two GWAS have been identified with possible links to OCD. The International OCD Foundation Genetics Collaborative (IOCDF-GC) and OCD Collaborative Genetics Association Studies (OCGAS) discovered a specific area on chromosome 12 demonstrated the strongest association with OCD, in a study involving 1465 cases and the analysis of over 410 autosomal and 9657 X chromosomal single nucleotide polymorphisms (IOCDF-GC and OCGAS 2018). Mattheisen et al. (2015) published a study that examined over 1065 families. Within these families, 1406 members had OCD and displayed a marker on chromosome 9, which has a strong association with the condition. A further meta-analysis reviewing both of these large studies found 15 potential genes involved in OCD, 12 of which were common between the studies. This groundbreaking research has significant implications for our understanding of OCD. It also has significant implications for newly recognised disorders that overlap and share the same genetic information located in the same area. Conditions hypothesised to be related include Tourette syndrome, tics, autism spectrum disorder, anorexia nervosa and the genetic diseases Prader-Willi syndrome and Angelman syndrome (Fornaro et al. 2009).

The GWAS found just over ten years ago confirm the twin studies of the 1930s, showing OCD as truly a mix of genetic and environmental factors. Unfortunately, the data available is predominantly of European ancestry and male-focused. Thus more research is required to explore the presentation and genetic coding of OCD in women, those of different ethnicities, and perinatal OCD (Samuels 2009).

Mother Nature or nurture? Environmental factors influencing OCD

The genetic understanding of OCD presents an exciting prospect for our comprehension and treatment of the condition. However, it is widely recognised that OCD is, at best, a combination of genetic predisposition and environmental influences that do not directly cause the disorder but rather increase vulnerability to developing the condition. Very little is known about the specific way in which environmental factors can increase the risk of OCD. However, the various factors listed below have been discussed in the evidence-based literature (Brander et al. 2016; Nasiri, Czuzoj-Shulman, & Abenhaim 2021):

- beta haemolytic streptococcal infections
- traumatic brain injury
- rheumatic fever
- prenatal/perinatal obstetric complications, including excessive maternal weight gain during pregnancy
- smoking in pregnancy
- history of trauma, including sexual, emotional, and physical abuse
- post-traumatic stress disorder
- birth trauma and complications
- significant life events.[1]

PERINATAL OCD AND HORMONES

In clinical practice, I frequently receive questions about whether perinatal OCD and other perinatal mental health issues are influenced by female hormones. It's a well-known fact that many women experience an increase in mental health concerns during pregnancy and in the postnatal period, along with mood fluctuations tied to their menstrual cycle. This occurs due to the intricate balance of hormones affecting both the womb and the brain. While research on the relationship between female hormones and OCD is still in its early stages, there is a sense of optimism about discovering potential connections. In this section, I summarise some of the evidence around the possible link between hormones and OCD in women.

In the past few years promising research surrounding the relationship between OCD and female hormones has been published. Mathes et al. (2019) noted that gender may play a part in the emergence of OCD symptoms in childhood and early adult life, but not necessarily

1 Some evidence of a link between traumatic life events and development of postnatal OCD in the mother exists. However, the limited research into the effects of the listed environmental factors pertains to foetal risk/child risk for developing OCD, not to risk to the mother for developing OCD.

impacting treatment outcome. Females were more likely to experience the onset of OCD at the time when they started having periods, and through life may notice a pattern of increased intensity of OCD symptoms just before and/or during their period (like mood changes when pre-menstrual). Some studies have shown worsening OCD at key hormonal moments in a woman's life – menarche, pregnancy, and postnatal specifically. No studies suggest a worsening of symptoms at the onset of or during menopause.

One hypothesis about differences in female lifespan suggests that ovarian sex hormones significantly influence the development of the disorder, putting females at higher risk for OCD during crucial life stages. A neuroendocrine research group in Canada investigated which specific hormones may participate in these fluctuations. Notably, oestrogen is believed to function in two ways: first, by enhancing serotonin activity in the brain; and second, by acting directly as a 'neuro-protective' agent. Serotonin is associated with mood improvement and the symptoms of OCD. Naturally, oestrogen levels decrease during menstruation, lower gradually through pregnancy, and sharply drop after childbirth. This reduction might be linked to heightened instances of perinatal OCD during these periods (Karpinski, Mattina, & Steiner 2017). Other studies indicate that individuals with OCD exhibit elevated plasma levels of the 'love hormone' oxytocin. This raises the question of whether the rise in oxytocin experienced during labour and breastfeeding could also play a role in the onset or exacerbation of perinatal OCD symptoms (Green & Graham 2022; Weiss et al. 1995). Currently, no research has specifically evaluated hormone levels alongside perinatal OCD symptoms, hindering the ability to draw robust conclusions about their correlation. Further studies are necessary in this field, especially regarding the potential impact of hormone replacement therapy on treating OCD in women during the perinatal phase.

So far, we have discussed the scientific basis of perinatal OCD in detail, from promising genetic findings to the significant influence of reproductive hormones during pregnancy and postnatally. In the next chapter, I adopt a psychodynamic approach, examining perinatal OCD through the lens of attachment theory and parenting styles – a topic of particular interest to new parents and a common question in clinical practice.

CHAPTER 9

Perinatal OCD and Attachment

I recently met a 22-year-old mother of four, who ticked all the boxes for perinatal OCD. She had experienced anxiety and OCD symptoms since childhood and had been known to child and adolescent mental health services (CAMHS) for most of her teen years. Throughout that time, she had been medicated for mixed depression and anxiety.

In our first hour of meeting, she told me all the symptoms that had been troubling her, namely around fear of harm coming to her and the children. When in the car, she would have horrific intrusive thoughts as well as visual 'flash-forwards' of an accident happening. When at home, her worries plagued her from the minute she woke up to the minute she put the children to bed; everything from worrying about a gas leak in the kitchen to the children drowning in the paddling pool. Even at night, she could not 'clock out' from her obsessional ruminations. She described patrolling her children's bedrooms through the night like a prison guard, checking their chest movements for breathing and ensuring the blanket didn't go over her toddler's head for fear of suffocation.

Although we did not go into detail, I was aware that my patient had had a difficult childhood. Both her parents were alcoholics, and she experienced a lot of emotional and physical abuse growing up with them. When she had her first child at 15, she dropped out of school. She was currently single but had some support from her ex-partner. Despite being tiny and frail in her frame, she displayed a strength and resilience beyond her years.

At the end of the appointment, I always ask if a patient has any questions for me. I did not, however, expect the profound question this young woman asked me: *'Doctor, honestly – why am I like this? Is there something wrong with me, or is it because of my bad childhood?'*

After a pause, I reassured her that there was nothing 'wrong' with her and told her I had had patients with the most stable upbringing who had suffered just as badly with anxiety and OCD symptoms. I explained to her about the 'you've got mail' neurobiological understandings of OCD we discussed in Chapter 8. She found the science helpful for understanding why she experienced these obsessional ruminations. However, her question got me thinking about the psychological and psychoanalytical underpinnings of the disorder. Specifically, I began to reflect on the origins of attachment styles and parenting styles, and how this can have a profound impact not only on our personality but also on how we relate to others, not to mention our mental health as adults.

Research has shown that the first year of a child's life is crucial. An infant's relationship with their caregiver during this critical time will lay the foundations of lifelong patterns of emotional attachment and relationship dynamics. A baby knows the intricacies of their caregivers' relational styles as early as seven months old and will adjust themselves to mirror the attachment to the individuals providing their care (HM Government 2021).

In this chapter, we will examine the psychological principles of OCD and attachment styles. These are important topics in discussing perinatal OCD, as this period highlights the parent–infant relationship. It is a broad area, and many books have been written about it. The brief overview I provide, however, presents the evidence base in the context of parenting and OCD.

ATTACHMENT THEORY

Interest in attachment theory grew in the mid-20th century, as did our hunger for cognitive and experimental psychology, moving away from earlier psychoanalytical thinking. This mirrored the clinical shift from focusing on the individual to the influence of the family unit on mental wellbeing, and in particular the mother playing a fundamental role, as we discussed earlier in Chapter 6. Mary Ainsworth created the 'strange situation' experiment in 1970, to understand the attachment styles of infants to their caregivers, and the principles of its findings continue to be used in clinical practice today. During the experiment, the mother left the room, and a stranger entered. Babies displayed three distinct responses, which led to the development of what we now recognise as attachment styles: secure, avoidant, and ambivalent (Ainsworth & Bell 1970).

The most common attachment style was secure attachment. A baby showed signs of distress when the mother left the room but felt joy when she returned. In avoidant attachment, the child exhibited extreme distress and was inconsolable even when the mother returned. In ambivalent attachment, the child showed no clear preference for the mother or the stranger. Ainsworth hypothesised that this could serve as an early protective mechanism to avoid rejection due to parental inconsistency. Later studies uncovered a fourth style: disorganised attachment. In this style, the baby displayed a range of unexpected reactions, including freezing or jerky movements. These children were thought to be at high risk of maternal neglect and abuse. These subsequent studies also suggested that challenges faced in early childhood could lead to behavioural and emotional difficulties later in life (Gagliardi 2021; Pederson et al. 2014).

Measuring attachment

As our understanding of attachment deepened, so did our ability to measure it in both children and adults. The Infant Care Index, created by Patricia Crittenden in the 1970s, offers a quick yet robust analysis based on a short video interaction between mother and baby. It can be used from birth up to approximately 15 months and has been widely employed in both research and clinical settings, especially as a screening tool for children involved in social-care proceedings related to children and families (Crittenden 2005).

Recent years have seen an increase in the use of video observations both in enhancing our understanding of parent–child attachment and as a form of clinical intervention. Examples include the Video Interactive Positive Parenting (VIPP) technique, Video Interactive Guidance (VIG), and the Parent–Infant

Interaction Observation Scale (PIIOS). More and more, community perinatal mental health services are adopting these innovative therapeutic methods to improve bonding and attachment between mothers and their children. They are relatively easy to understand for both clinicians and patients and have become popular interventions, providing positive reinforcement or acting as a natural deterrent from undesirable behaviours to strengthen the mother–child relationship. Participants describe feeling comfortable being recorded on a mobile device or tablet, especially as many mothers and babies are now familiar with and accustomed to digital media (O'Hara et al. 2019).

The Adult Attachment Interview (AAI), devised in 1984, remains the most popular and scientifically validated method for obtaining a detailed analysis of adult attachment styles. The semi-structured interview, however, requires both time and skill. It can take over an hour to complete, even longer to transcribe and analyse, and must be administered by a trained clinician to avoid false outcomes.

LIMITATIONS

Attachment theory has, for the most part, been ingrained into the psychodynamic psyche, so to speak, without much challenge, until recently. Early researchers in the field did not address the phenomenon of potential intergenerational transmission of attachment styles (e.g. 'like mother, like daughter'). They also did not consider that both attachment to the caregiver and the development of personality occur, arguably, on a continuum until the child reaches school age, with three distinct phases: 2–6 months, 6–24 months, and 2–6 years. Personally, I feel that even this is too simplistic, as it does not account for other important influences outside this narrow time frame. Clinically, we know that a lot happens physically, psychologically, and emotionally for the mother and child in the first eight weeks of life before the GP postnatal check-up. Parents of older children will know all too well that attachment continues to develop well into the teenage and early adult years. Over this period, both the parent and child change as individuals, as does their relationship to each other along with the situations they face, together and apart. External factors, such as the birth of additional siblings, parental separation, starting school, and death in the family, may also influence the attachment relationship.

OCD AND PARENTING STYLES

Child development psychologist Diane Baumrind first described parenting style in the 1960s. In keeping with the thinking of the time, her work emphasised maternal bonding and attachment as being 'responsible' for the development of mental health conditions in children. It also gave heightened attention to the influence parenting styles had on children's behaviours, for better or worse. Baumrind described three main parenting styles believed to be the blueprint influencing children's personal qualities (Baumrind 1966).

- *The permissive parent* seeks to behave in a non-confrontational and positive manner towards the child's impulses, desires, and actions. She (the parent) discusses decisions with him (the child) and provides explanations for family rules. She makes few demands on her child and presents herself as their equal, without guiding or influencing their behaviour. She allows the child to regulate their activities as much as possible, avoids exercising control, and does not encourage them to obey externally imposed standards.

- *The authoritarian parent*, in contrast, tries to shape and control the child's behaviour and attitudes according to a set standard of conduct, often aligned with a higher authority such as their religious beliefs. She (the parent) prioritises parental obedience and opts for forceful measures to suppress the child's self-will based on her beliefs about what is right. She is hesitant to debate the pros and cons with a child, believing that the child should accept her word as the truth to be obeyed.

- *The authoritative parent* attempts to guide the child's activities in a rational, issue-focused manner. She (the parent) encourages verbal discussion and shares with the child the reasoning

> behind her policies. This parenting style falls somewhere between permissive and authoritarian. The parent maintains firm control when necessary but avoids being overly restrictive. As the adult, she assumes responsibility and leadership while recognising and respecting the child's individual interests.

Discussion about parenting styles may seem outdated. However, there remains a focus on how parenting influences children. Some might argue this is a form of 'rebranding', especially with the rise of social media providing a portal into understanding different family dynamics and practices. Patients at our clinic often find themselves torn between advice on child-focused 'gentle/baby-led parenting' practices, popularised by American actress and educator Janet Lansbury,[1] and 'parent-led parenting', promoted by maternity nurse and author Gina Ford.[2]

Regarding perinatal OCD, the evidence about parenting styles is lacking. We recognise there may be anxiety about this issue on two fronts: whether the mother with perinatal OCD developed the condition due to her own parents' upbringing of her, and whether she might unintentionally put her child at risk of developing it as a side effect of her parenting behaviours – possibly overcautious or neglectful if preoccupied with OCD.

Of course, the discussion is somewhat more complex than a simple A + B = C hypothesis. Alonso et al. (2004) recognise that developing OCD will not only affect an individual's quality of life but may also place strain on the entire family unit, potentially leading to changes in parenting style and relationship dynamics. As parents become involved in their child's mental health needs, their responses may vary (e.g. rejection, criticism, overprotection, or reassurance). This, in turn, may reinforce the obsessive-compulsive cycle discussed in Chapter 5, mainly to avoid confrontation. However, it is difficult to determine whether this influences OCD development in adulthood. Behavioural theorists suggest that social learning, especially within the parent–child relationship, may also contribute to OCD development in those who are 'biologically vulnerable'. Nevertheless, the influence

1 See www.janetlansbury.com
2 See www.ginaford.com

of parental behaviours on the emergence of obsessive-compulsive symptoms or OCD remains inconclusive (Alonso et al. 2004).

The experience of perinatal OCD is not only shaped by our individual and familial experiences but also influenced by the systemic factors around us. In the next chapter, I explore how aspects of society, such as being in an ethnic minority or part of the queer community, may impact not only our wellbeing but also accessibility to mental healthcare. I also reflect on the care of fathers during the perinatal period, advocating for better support for partners during this vulnerable time.

CHAPTER 10

Thinking Outside the Box

Seeing Perinatal OCD from the Perspective of Non-Dominant Communities

So far in the book, I have predominantly addressed perinatal OCD from the perspective of the cis-heteronormative and racial-normative viewpoint. We know, however, in clinical practice that our patient population is extremely diverse and there are several cultural and social factors that may influence both the maternity experience and that of mental illness in the perinatal period. In this chapter, I will explore important aspects of perinatal OCD presentation in Black and ethnic minorities and in the lesbian, gay, bisexual, transgender and queer identifying (LGBTQ+) community. I will also discuss how religion and spirituality may influence perinatal OCD (separate from the OCD theme of SCRUPULOSITY discussed in Chapter 3). This chapter provides an overview of these topics and an invitation to explore further through personal study and shared learning in your workplace and communities.

PERINATAL OCD IN BLACK, ASIAN, AND ETHNIC MINORITY GROUPS

A lot has been written in recent years around both the maternal and mental health inequalities and discrimination faced by those of Black, Asian, and minority ethnicities (BAME). Unfortunately, relatively little information exists for OCD experienced by these minority groups, let alone those who are expecting and/or have children.

Historically, clinical research trials into both physical and mental health issues have lacked true ethnic representation of the population. Consequently, there has been limited information on how treatment might be effective in these groups or how it could cause adverse side effects. Mental health practitioners in the US and the UK have been taking measures to close these knowledge gaps. In 1994, the National Institutes of Health in the US first published the *Outreach Notebook for the NIH Guidelines on the Inclusion of Women and Minorities as Subjects in Clinical Research*. This policy required the inclusion of women and minorities in all NIH-funded clinical research unless there was a strong reason to justify their exclusion.[1] Recently, Channel 4 in the UK aired 'The Black Maternity Scandal', an episode of the documentary series *Dispatches* discussing the disadvantages faced by Black and Asian women regarding their maternity experiences and birth outcomes (Shannon 2021), as highlighted in a recent position statement by the Royal College of Obstetricians and Gynaecologists (n.d.). The statistics, when viewed clearly, are shocking:

- Black women are at a fourfold increased risk of dying during labour and in the year following childbirth compared to white women.
- Asian women are at a twofold risk of dying during labour or in the year following childbirth.
- Black and Asian women are more likely to have a medicalised birth with hospital intervention.
- Ethnic minorities are more at risk of developing conditions such as diabetes, high blood pressure, and obesity, all of which have the potential to affect pregnancy and delivery.

The potential influence of systemic racism within the NHS, especially regarding how women are assessed, examined, or referred based on unconscious bias, presents a troubling reality (Five X More 2024).

1 Updated information on the policy can be found at https://grants.nih.gov/policy-and-compliance/policy-topics/inclusion/women-and-minorities/guideline

MENTAL HEALTH MATTERS IN THE PERINATAL PERIOD

The MBRRACE-UK (2025) report examines the causes of maternal deaths within a year of childbirth, identifying mental health as one of the top five contributors. It also highlights that women from Black, Asian, and other ethnic minority backgrounds face greater social disadvantages – including higher rates of domestic violence, poorer housing and socio-economic conditions, increased substance use, and a higher risk of mental health problems.

No woman in the 21st century should die in the year following childbirth, especially not in a leading developed nation at the forefront of medical excellence and technological innovation such as the UK. It is vital to recognise a correlation that many have overlooked: women are dying after childbirth due to mental health issues, and women of colour are also dying related to maternal outcomes. Although there is limited literature in this area, we can gather key principles from related research. We know that women of colour are less likely to seek help for their mental health issues and have reduced access to healthcare compared to others, despite the NHS being a free service available to all (Hoang et al. 2022; Hoang et al. 2023, Spurlock & Pickler 2024; Williams et al. 2010). Common barriers faced by women of Black, Asian, and other ethnic minorities when accessing mental health or maternity care include:

- language and communication challenges
- difficulties navigating institutional policies (particularly during the COVID-19 pandemic)
- familial pressures
- experiences of shame and blame
- dismissal of pain and withholding of treatment
- stigma surrounding mental illness and accepting professional help.

In addition to these barriers, some women who have immigrated to the UK from other countries may have limited understanding of mental health conditions such as OCD, as mental health may not have been discussed or taught in their country of origin. I have cared for many such women who, with the help of an interpreter, have told me that 'this is just how I have always been'.

It is important to recognise, however, that patterns of reluctance to access mental health services are not confined to those who have moved abroad. Children of immigrants may grow up facing the complexities of intersectional discrimination (co-occurring racism and gender-based discrimination). Often, they are raised in a family and/or cultural setting that may minimise the importance of mental and emotional health and wellbeing. These families often prioritise educational achievement and financial security. Women, in particular, may face additional conflicting messages about conforming to traditional ideas and expectations of marriage, family, and gender roles, as previously discussed in Chapter 4 (Ahn et al. 2022; Forbes, Yang, & Lim 2023).

In 2024, the Kaiser Family Foundation, a US-based nonprofit organisation specialising in health issues and health policy analysis across the US and globally, examined racial disparities in maternal and infant health following COVID-19 (Hill et al. 2024). They found that the pre-existing challenges faced by Black and ethnic minority families had worsened. Underlying social and economic inequalities were deeply rooted in a history and culture characterised by ongoing racism and discrimination. Noted challenges included:

- access to food security and healthier food options
- social integration
- increased exposure to violence and trauma
- poorer housing and unemployment alongside rising debt and medical bills.

Together, these challenges impacted not only on general health and wellbeing but the ability to access safe and appropriate maternity care.

Although statistics indicate that OCD affects individuals from different backgrounds equally, ethnic minorities with OCD are underrepresented in research and clinical settings. Fernández de la Cruz et al. (2016) completed a community survey of nearly 300 Black and ethnic minority parents living in South London regarding their understanding and beliefs about OCD. They discovered that those of Indian heritage were more likely to minimise OCD, believing it to be a mild mental health condition and displaying ambivalence towards seeking help or starting treatment. Conversely, individuals of Black African and Black Caribbean origin were more likely to struggle with recognising OCD and knowing where to find assistance. They also expressed greater concerns about experiencing discrimination within the NHS, feelings of mistrust towards the medical system, and a preference for seeking counsel from religious leaders.

CULTURAL AND RELIGIOUS CONSIDERATIONS FOR PERINATAL OCD

As discussed previously, understanding a patient's cultural background and upbringing is important in the assessment and management of a woman's transition to motherhood, and their experiences of mental illness during the perinatal period. Culture can be defined as the values, beliefs, and practices related to a specific ethnocultural group that are passed down through generations (Betancourt & López 1993). Cultural experiences and expectations shape the way we understand and interpret pregnancy, the birth experience, the division of baby-care and other labour, and our relationship with the baby. Cultural factors influence how we think, behave, and process information about the world around us, which often determines specific actions and behaviours within individuals, families, and the wider community. Even our knowledge and beliefs about mental health, and the associated stigmas surrounding seeking help during the perinatal period, can be influenced by what we have been brought up to believe is 'normal' or 'the right way'. For some, this may relate to strong cultural or family values. For others, it may be rooted in their religious beliefs.

Although I merge religion and culture in this chapter, I understand in clinical practice that the very concept of identity and belonging is shaped by complex and diverse relationships. For example, people may be born and raised in the UK, but their family could originate from a foreign country which also displays considerable internal diversity in beliefs and practices. One might say they are Indian, for instance, but India is not a monolith – it has many provinces, languages, foods, religions, and a caste system. Today, it is also common for families to be blended, with partners from different cultural backgrounds sharing numerous cultural customs. Religious and/or cultural differences can be a source of tension or difficulty during the perinatal period, especially if there is a clash around traditional practices for a newborn between the families, or if one family's understanding of mental health or gender roles differs from the other.

Several studies have explored the link between OCD and religion. As discussed in Chapter 3, RELIGIOUS OCD, or SCRUPULOSITY, is characterised by excessive concerns about religious details and the person's morality. Obsessions may appear as persistent doubts and fears of punishment from God for being a 'sinful' person. Compulsions can include repetitive prayers, religious rituals, and seeking reassurance. Higher rates of OCD are observed in countries adhering to Jewish and Islamic faith, and they are more likely to experience religion-based obsessions. In Egypt, 60% of individuals with OCD report having religious obsessions; in Saudi Arabia, 50%, and in Israel, 50%. Researchers in Baltimore, US, have found that although religion seems to be one arena where OCD can manifest, it is not a determinant of the disorder (Nicolini et al. 2017).

Themes surrounding OCD can blend religious, ethical, and moral beliefs, aligning with teachings found in religious scripture and practice. For instance, experiencing 'Catholic guilt' and the urge for confession might obscure the distinction between illness and normal religious behaviour during OCD episodes, as well as during the perinatal period through feelings of maternal guilt and shame. In the Jewish faith, rituals are central to teachings and practices, which may offer a space for individuals with OCD to express their symptoms without fear of judgement, or their symptoms (such as compulsively praying repeatedly) can be disguised as 'heightened devotion'. As Yasmin's case vignette, discussed in Chapter 3, illustrates, RELIGIOUS OCD themes can become entangled with FEAR OF CONTAMINATION OCD themes, centred on the dual concepts of being 'pure' and 'clean' both hygienically and morally/spiritually (Nedeljkovic et al. 2012). When these overlap in clinical practice, involving faith leaders is crucial to support the treatment and management plan (Greenberg & Shefler 2008).

Superstitions and OCD

Superstition is another intriguing belief model common in ancient and modern societies. It blurs the boundaries between obsessions and magical thinking, which can be seen not only in OCD, but in personality and psychotic disorders.

Despite the technological advances and the wealth of scientific information available to us, superstitious beliefs and practices continue to thrive. Pregnancy attracts a variety of beliefs and superstitious recommendations for expectant parents. These include caution about receiving gifts before the baby's arrival or eating certain foods believed to bring bad luck.

At the core of superstition lies the need to feel a sense of control and self-efficacy, especially when under stress. For the majority, having superstitious thoughts is integrated into their psyche and coping strategies and is deemed acceptable within cultural norms. The key difference is this: in those with superstitious and/or religious beliefs, engaging in this sphere offers comfort; in individuals with OCD exhibiting religious and superstitious symptoms, their engagement stems mainly from fear (if I do not do X, something terrible will happen to me or my loved ones). Such engagement causes significant anxiety, and compulsive behaviours are employed to neutralise these emotions.

Although it is arguable that superstitious behaviours are performed due to a fear of something bad happening, the intensity is not as severe as in a clinical condition. The section on RELIGIOUS OCD in Chapter 3 has more on this.

IT'S COMPLICATED: PERINATAL OCD IN FATHERS, SAME-SEX PARTNERS, AND THE LGBTQ+ COMMUNITY[2]

The birth of a new baby almost inevitably brings changes to the entire family, not just the mother. Like a stone thrown into a pond, the impact of a newborn ripples through the family, affecting parents, grandparents, siblings, and others. In most cases, expanding

2 In this section, I will not be discussing the issue of obsessional fears around intrusive thoughts of a sexual nature (e.g. homosexuality). This was discussed in Chapter 2.

the family is a celebration, filled with new hope and regarded as a generally positive life event. However, fathers and partners may also struggle with the adjustment to having a baby and may experience a range of emotions as they navigate the early years with their partner. The impact of these changes may be more noticeable in partners who are cohabiting but can also manifest through challenges faced when parenting separately (Walker, Blackie, & Nedeljkovic 2021).

Over the past decade, awareness and recognition of the challenges fathers face regarding their mental health during the perinatal period have increased. One study reported that most fathers describe becoming a father as a most wonderful and defining experience, one associated with feelings of love, pride, and improvement in their relationships. The same study also discussed how this time of intense change could bring about new mental health concerns or worsen pre-existing ones (Bradley & Slade 2011).

As we know, obsessive-compulsive symptoms are common in new parents and do not necessarily indicate the development of a disorder. OCD, however, is a prevalent mental illness that affects males and females equally and does not discriminate based on sexual orientation. It is quite possible that a non-birthing partner has experienced OCD in the past or is currently struggling with symptoms that may intensify with the upcoming arrival. This can manifest in various ways, but, like with the mother, it primarily involves a fear of harm coming to the baby. Researchers have described fathers as being susceptible to perinatal OCD, and that becoming a parent may trigger intrusive thoughts and fears, such as questioning *'Am I a good Dad?'* or *'What if I really am a child molester?'* Fathers may also experience intrusive 'flash-forward' violent and distressing images, such as shaking babies to death or causing accidental harm to the baby, or a compulsive need to protect their partner and infant with feelings of inflated responsibility (Abramowitz et al. 2003a; Walker et al. 2021).

Risk factors for fathers/partners experiencing mental health difficulties include:

- early negative experiences (including coming to terms with their own experience of being parented and/or childhood abuse)

- stressful life events, such as work pressures, financial insecurity, or redundancy
- coping with changes in the relationship (particularly the needs of a newborn adding another person into the mix).

Having a smaller support network has also been shown to have a negative impact on both father's/partner's mental health and the health of the relationship in managing the challenges of the early years. Further concerns a father/partner may experience include pressure around being able to financially support their growing family, as well as adjusting to the new roles they have (such as their partner, who was previously working, now being on maternity leave) (Walker et al. 2021).

Although UK government legislation has recently changed to promote equality in parental leave, many men may still feel hesitant to request extended leave from work. They might fear the stigma of taking a career break, which could jeopardise their job security and make them feel at risk of redundancy. Currently, most corporate and public sector organisations offer fathers/partners a discretionary two-week paternity leave; however, I have encountered many fathers/partners who have felt unable to take time off after having a baby, which will inevitably affect their parenting.

INVISIBLE MEN

Other systemic or organisational factors may affect a father's mental health. For example, services within the perinatal mental health and maternity setting tend to be biased towards women. I have met many fathers who have described feeling 'invisible' in antenatal clinics and in the labour room. They report not even being given eye contact, let alone the opportunity to ask questions or the support to process what they are seeing and hearing (e.g. witnessing a traumatic birth). Sadly, services continue to let fathers/partners down by offering support only for mothers or only providing support during working hours when the father/partner might find it difficult to attend.

In perinatal mental health services, we are actively working to address this bias by making our services more inclusive of men and partners and recognising that either parent can experience mental health difficulties during the perinatal period. We regularly hold joint perinatal sessions with fathers and partners (with the patient's consent) and organise meetings, such as pre-birth planning sessions, where birthing partners can be present. NHS England's long-term plan focuses on improving the family's wellbeing as a whole (Department of Health and Social Care 2025a), meaning that partners will now be offered screening and/or assessment of their own mental health if they are struggling during or after the birth.

However, seeking support can cause stigma for everyone, including partners. The way men present mental health needs may differ from that of women (specifically, they are more likely to increase alcohol consumption or use illicit substances).

Statistics also indicate a higher risk of domestic violence and abuse during a woman's pregnancy and postnatal period. This may relate to fathers managing their own mental health issues or the need for control during the perinatal phase. The risk of domestic violence or abuse can also be significant for the child, requiring safeguarding protocols. The paper *'The Myth of Invisible Men'* presents evidence about serious incidents of babies under one year old being harmed or killed by their father (Child Safeguarding Practice Review Panel 2021). The paper acknowledges the needs of fathers, who may have had difficult childhoods and struggle to manage their emotions or mental health. These fathers tend to have lower levels of distress tolerance and may sometimes express themselves through anger and violence (often under the influence of substances). The report highlights that suicide is also the leading cause of death among men aged 25 to 65, which is the same age range for fatherhood.

Our aim should be to recognise that fathers and partners are also vulnerable to worsening OCD and mental health difficulties during the perinatal period. Services can improve access for fathers and partners to support with their own mental health, whether in primary care or psychiatric settings. The engagement of fathers must be integrated into current and future programmes such as family hubs, the Supporting Families Programme, and follow-up work to the Leadsom Report into the first 1000 days (HM Government 2021).

SHARED MOTHERHOOD: PERINATAL OCD IN THE LGBTQ+ COMMUNITY

Sexual and gender minorities (individuals that identify outside of the gender-normative cis-male cis-female and heteronormative 'straight' mainstream) experience stressors that increase risk for psychiatric disorders. Although the research is limited in this area, there is already clear evidence that the lesbian, gay, and bisexual communities have elevated risks of emotional dysregulation, mental illness, and anxiety compared with the general population. A recent study also notes that they are also up to nine times more likely to be diagnosed or receive treatment for OCD (Bezahler et al. 2024)

The LGBTQ+ community is increasingly vulnerable to discrimination, rejection, prejudice, and internalised homophobia. Females in same-sex relationships experience higher rates of depression, anxiety, sexual violence, and sexual coercion. They are also at greater risk of becoming victims of physical and sexual violence, social isolation during specific experiences such as the perinatal period, and suicidal behaviours (Agardh et al. 2022; Pinciotti et al. 2022).

Despite higher rates of OCD, more psychiatric comorbidities, and minority stressors, little is known about the clinical presentation and treatment outcomes of gender minorities with OCD. Same-sex, trans, and non-binary couples may also face an additional challenge of psychological stress involved in assisted conception. Over the past 20 years, changes in attitudes and law towards lesbian and gay couples, as well as the expansion of criteria for assisted conception techniques such as in-vitro fertilisation (IVF) or intra-uterine insemination (IUI), have made assisted reproduction treatment more accepted and accessible.

In the UK, the right to civil partnership for same-sex couples was recognised in 2004, and same-sex marriage was introduced in 2014. In 2008, the Human Fertilisation and Embryology Act was amended to reflect the legal changes, by removing previous requirements for 'a child's need for a father', thus allowing female partners to become legal parents. Around the same time, equality legislation outlawed discrimination based on protected characteristics and prohibited refusal of fertility treatment based on sexual orientation. Shared motherhood IVF treatment is becoming increasingly accepted among assisted reproductive technique practitioners and patients in Europe (Bodri et al. 2018).

Despite the legal and social recognition that same-sex, trans, and non-binary people are becoming parents, invisibility continues to persist in public health policy, starting with the language we use. Terms such as 'maternal mental health' and 'paternal mental health' reflect cis-heteronormativity. While primary care, maternity, and mental health services aim to provide holistic, individualised care, for many in these marginalised communities this is far from the collective experience. Individuals have reported feeling isolated in their perinatal journey, feeling 'not man enough, not trans enough, not pregnant enough, and not safe enough during pregnancy, birth, and the postpartum' (Greenfield & Darwin 2021). Further inclusive research involving LGBTQ+ participation is needed to inform future service design. A simple, positive change all services involved with families in the perinatal period can implement is to start recording sexual orientation and gender (in all its forms) as part of routine demographic data. Hearing the voices of the LGBTQ+ community in perinatal mental health research would foster a dialogue to uncover potential inequalities that previously remained hidden due to lack of recording and detection. Services may then be adapted to meet local needs to improve outcomes for all parents and families (Kerppola et al. 2019).

To summarise, health professionals should keep in mind the diverse experiences of perinatal OCD in marginalised communities and have increased vigilance and awareness that those from BAME and LGBTQ+ communities may not have equitable access to perinatal mental healthcare. Fathers and partners may also be vulnerable to developing symptoms of OCD and mental illness during this time. In Part 4, we shift our attention to making an accurate diagnosis of perinatal OCD. I provide a helpful checklist of sample questions for a thorough assessment of OCD presenting in pregnancy and postnatal, as well as supporting information on differential diagnoses.

PART 4

DIAGNOSING PERINATAL OCD

In Part 4, I provide a detailed analysis on the assessment and diagnosis of OCD presenting in the perinatal period. This part provides practical insights to support the clinician, such as helpful open questions to ask in assessments, and consideration of mental health law and safeguarding. I also provide an overview of differential diagnoses to keep in mind. My aim is to illuminate specific conditions that share similar characteristics with perinatal OCD and that may be confused or misdiagnosed in clinical practice.

CHAPTER 11

Understanding the Barriers to Diagnosing Perinatal OCD and Relevant Mental Health Law

As discussed in Part I, we know that perinatal OCD is under-detected and under-diagnosed. Before we delve into the assessment and diagnosis of perinatal OCD, it is worth reflecting on the barriers (both personal and systemic) that women and families face in being referred to specialist perinatal mental health services.

BARRIERS TO DIAGNOSIS

Several barriers hinder the detection, diagnosis, and treatment of perinatal OCD. Consider Chloe's story (below). On the surface, her condition seems to be a straightforward concern about her baby's health. In reality, it is more complex.

CASE VIGNETTE – CHLOE

Chloe is a young, first-time mother. She trained as a hairdresser but became pregnant in her final year and was not able to complete her qualification. She told me, however, that she didn't mind, as she has always wanted children, and she and her boyfriend,

Callum, of two years were excited about welcoming their first child (and the first grandchild on both sides of the family).

Chloe's pregnancy and labour were documented as 'unremarkable' in her hospital records, indicating all was 'normal' and uncomplicated. She described feeling 'both terrified and excited' about being a mum. She left for home the day after her delivery with lots of support from her partner and family, who live close by. They were on hand to help with the whirlwind of the newborn period.

Chloe was referred to our service by her health visitor, who expressed concerns that Chloe was 'very anxious' about the baby in the weeks following the birth. Chloe noted that she had been feeling very anxious since her son was born, worrying that something might happen to him. When I asked her to elaborate, she could not say what exactly she was worried about, only that he might fall ill, get hurt, or die. She also described feeling anxious about her son's breathing. She reported getting up every hour of the night, checking on him to see if he was okay. She also got anxious about room temperature and kept a room thermometer in every room, which she checked regularly.

Chloe lived in a flat on the top floor of her apartment block. She avoided leaving the flat, petrified she might accidentally drop the baby down the stairs. Her health visitor had discussed with her the wealth of support services available in her local community, including breastfeeding drop-in clinics, baby sensory classes and baby massage. Chloe described the idea of attending any of these services 'overwhelming', preferring telephone appointments or home visits where possible. Chloe disclosed that she spent her nights awake, even though the baby slept relatively well. She often was 'googling into the early hours' about everything and anything to do with baby illnesses.

On our first appointment, Chloe's son Max lit up the room. He was a happy child with a wide, toothless smile and full of energy. She informed me that she had never had any mental health issues previously. She had experienced bullying at school, for which she had seen a therapist for a few sessions in her teens, which she found helpful. She had experienced panic attacks in the past when under a lot of stress in a previous relationship but

> described her current partner as very supportive. She tried medication for anxiety three years ago, but quit after a couple of days as she felt it made her worse.

Patients with the kinds of symptoms described by Chloe rarely make it to the attention of their GP, let alone a specialist maternity mental health service. Her situation is one I have often encountered during my time working in mental health. Although Chloe's concerns started soon after delivery, the referral was made to perinatal mental health services months down the line. Patients like Chloe engage an arduous process to be seen by a perinatal psychiatrist, requiring a lot of bravery on the part of the patient. I have outlined below some of the barriers and loopholes that lead to a missed (or mistaken) diagnosis.

Barrier 1 – 'But it's normal'

Having a first child is a pivotal, life-changing moment for the mother and her whole family. In most cases, a child is welcomed into the world as a happy occasion with lots of excitement and hopes for a new generation. Choosing baby names, growing-bump selfies, attending antenatal classes, and shopping for adorable and impossibly tiny baby onesies make the experience joyful and one to remember. For the first-time mother, regardless of the books she has read or the advice asked of those who have 'been there, done that, got the (stained) t-shirt', nothing can prepare her for motherhood. Many feel that they just 'learn as you go along' with a 'winging it' attitude.

Bringing a baby into the world introduces new responsibilities. For many, this can cause anxiety and feel overwhelming – sometimes even 'terrifying', as Chloe described. The saying 'to worry is to be a mother' is common in many cultures. As discussed in Chapter 4, 'mother' signifies not just responsibility but also unconditional love, knowledge, and expertise in caring for children. Many still believe in 'mother's intuition', which remains influential in clinical settings nationwide – mothers often sense something is wrong with their child even if there are no obvious symptoms.

Many individuals normalise these feelings of doubt and worry, either through their own efforts – such as self-talk, minimising concerns, or overriding thoughts – or through reassurance from others. For first-time parents, worry is often viewed as natural and part of adjusting to parenthood. As a result, many obsessive thoughts and compulsive behaviours during early months of motherhood go unnoticed. Despite feeling that something is seriously wrong, patients are frequently reassured by loved ones and professionals that their experiences are normal and expected.

With perinatal OCD, we also see an obsessional, inflated sense of maternal responsibility coupled with fear of something seriously bad happening to the child. Family and friends might also collude with the patient; for example, encouraging the nocturnal googling or the constant checking, in the hope that these behaviours will ease their anxieties, allowing them to 'relax'. Sadly, however, as we see repeatedly in the case of perinatal OCD, this is rarely the case. Instead, it just adds fuel to the flames.

Barrier 2 – It's not a 'real' mental illness

Many patients arrive late to our services because they believe what they are experiencing is not 'real' mental illness. They consider it less deserving of help and support compared to more high-profile conditions, such as postnatal depression or bipolar disorder. Recently, the public health message has been clear: individuals should be more proactive about their health and rely less on professional support, implying that only those who are 'seriously ill' have access to help. This is partly due to the pressure on frontline staff and services across all sectors, along with growing waiting lists. Those with perinatal OCD symptoms rarely have the knowledge, expertise, or perspective (other than subjective feeling) as to what is both 'serious' and/or an 'illness'. The patient with OCD understands their thoughts are 'ridiculous' or 'unreal'. This muddies the water around accessing specialist mental health support, particularly if the patient feels there is a 'hierarchy of need'.

Patients with OCD (both general and perinatal) are also often high-functioning individuals. They may be able to continue with their professional and personal life, to some extent, hidden and unscathed. Like Chloe, they are often well supported by family (although, as discussed earlier, this can be a double-edged sword), reducing the need for professional help, as the condition can be 'managed behind closed doors'. This is often the case with generalised OCD. However, we have seen both clinically and through research that those with OCD often relapse and/or get worse in the perinatal period. The added complexity of a newborn thrown into the mix makes it much harder to cope with the condition than it was previously (Abramovitch et al. 2010).

Barrier 3 – Lack of awareness

Asking for help for one's mental health can feel like asking for directions in a new town. Someone may know the destination the traveller is looking for and give the correct information to get them there. Someone else may know the destination but cannot explain how to get there correctly or in a way the traveller can comprehend. Others may not know the destination, but do not want to admit that they don't know so give vague directions that may or may not help.

It is not only the traveller that feels lost – unfortunately many health professionals do not feel adequately trained to recognise perinatal OCD. Sadly, perinatal OCD rarely makes it on the differential diagnosis – not just in primary and community care services but even in mental health services. Doctors, nurses, or midwives may look at a new mother and err on the side of reassurance, telling them that it will get better with time, or they may make dismissive statements such as 'If you think this is bad, just wait until the terrible twos!'

Barrier 4: Logistics

Access to perinatal services and treatments for conditions like perinatal OCD has greatly improved over the past five years. However, the reality remains that accessing services can be a postcode lottery. Despite significant government investment in improving mental health support for women and families as part of NHS England's long-term plan (Department of Health and Social Care 2025a), confusion persists among health professionals and patients about to whom and where patients should be referred for treatment. In my own area in London, I can identify 11 potential routes through which a patient with perinatal OCD could be seen and offered support:

- local primary care talking therapies
- their GP
- their primary care mental health team
- the community mental health team
- the perinatal community mental health team (within that is a CBT psychotherapist or parent–infant psychiatrist)

- online group therapy for mothers
- crisis home treatment team
- specialist perinatal mother and baby unit
- national perinatal OCD service
- national OCD and body dysmorphic disorder unit
- the specialist maternity psychology services or the new maternity services for those who have experienced obstetric trauma and/or baby loss.

Each service has its own distinct referral inclusion and exclusion criteria. While the communication between services is improving, it has a long way to go. The sad truth is there is a lot of pressure placed on GPs and other referring professionals to make the 'right' decision. Whatever decision is made will often dictate the future pathway of care, which has become more convoluted with the goalposts constantly changing. This has resulted in referrals not being made in the first place, as referrers feel ill equipped to know how or where to signpost.

Barrier 5: Missing the diagnosis and misdiagnosis

Before we can make a management plan, we need to be sure of our diagnosis. Often, perinatal OCD is not only missed as a diagnosis, but misdiagnosed as perinatal anxiety, depression, or even schizophrenia. This may be due, in part, to the patient's reluctance to disclose certain symptoms because they feel embarrassed or ashamed about what they feel (see Barrier 6 below). It could also be due to inadequate training in perinatal mental illnesses, let alone perinatal OCD, on the part of the clinician.

Mental health is a very limited component of clinical training. Doctors in the UK spend, on average, up to six weeks in a clinical psychiatry attachment during approximately six years of medical school. Of those six weeks, they would be lucky to spend even a day shadowing a perinatal mental health team; their exposure is very much dependent on the quality of the training programme and enthusiasm of educators to ensure perinatal mental health is integrated into the undergraduate curriculum. Sadly, should doctors specialise in GP or psychiatry, perinatal psychiatry remains an optional rotation.

However, change is on the horizon. The Royal Colleges of Psychiatrists, General Practitioners, and Obstetricians & Gynaecologists are working together with medical schools and training schemes across the country to ensure that perinatal mental health is included not only within the examination system but also through the introduction of taster weeks, student-selected components, and promoted training in perinatal psychiatry (Royal College of Psychiatrists 2021).

Barrier 6: Not wanting to be referred – stigma of mental illness in motherhood

Despite all the progress in education and the investment in perinatal mental health services nationwide, our services are only the tip of the iceberg. Beneath the surface lies a significant demand for support related to mental health in the perinatal period (and mental health in general). However, for numerous complex reasons, many people are hesitant to seek help. We recognise that stigma surrounding mental health remains a major barrier for many individuals. The additional layer of being labelled as a 'bad mother' intensifies this stigma. Edwards and Timmons (2005) found that stigma in motherhood was experienced both internally and externally. Themes of concern include:

- reluctance for disclosure
- varied access to services
- feelings of being a bad mother
- concerns about being labelled/diagnosed with a mental illness.

The significant gap in the study is all those who suffer in silence. Patients fear referral because they worry about what it will mean, not only from a psychological perspective (being possibly perceived as 'failing' as a mother), but also practically, with the genuine concern of 'my baby being taken away' (by social services). A universal criterion for referral to perinatal mental health services across the country is consent – a woman must be aware that the health professional wants to refer her for additional support. However, we receive many 'incomplete' referrals because the consent has not been obtained.

To summarise, barriers to accessing support for perinatal OCD are complex. They may start with concerns about stigma or minimising symptoms, and then extend to confusion about diagnosis, referral processes, and available help. In most cases, those experiencing perinatal OCD will have the mental capacity to understand their mental health needs and are able to make informed decisions about their treatment and management plan. In the next section, I will briefly summarise important aspects of UK mental health law should concerns be raised about mental capacity or the severity of the mental illness.

MENTAL CAPACITY, THE MENTAL HEALTH ACT, AND DEPRIVATION OF LIBERTY

The likelihood of a patient diagnosed with perinatal OCD encountering the law is low. However, it is important that all health professionals have some basic understanding of these matters. In this section, I briefly discuss the key principles for clinical practice regarding the Mental Health Act 1983, the Mental Capacity Act 2005, and safeguarding processes.[1] It is also worthwhile to note that at the time of writing this, a new Mental Health Bill has been introduced to the House of Commons in May 2025. The aim is to modernise the existing Mental Health Act. The Mental Health Act 1983 has undergone many revisions but remains the key legislation in the UK aimed at providing appropriate reception, care, and treatment for those with a mental disorder.

Mental Health Act 1983

The Mental Health Act provides a legal framework for care in the case of mental health disorders or disability of the mind. According to the law, individuals who are very unwell and/or may pose a risk to themselves or others can be brought into hospital or a place of safety for their assessment and treatment.

In cases of severe OCD, most patients needing hospital admission will agree with their treatment plan. When they do, they are classified as a 'voluntary' patient. This is a particularly important distinction. The psychological treatment of OCD cannot be forced on someone; it

1 The government is due to launch a consultation in 2026 on Liberty Protection Safeguards to improve safeguarding for vulnerable people (Department of Health and Social Care 2025b).

requires personal motivation and engagement in the therapeutic process. However, there may be rare circumstances where the patient's severe OCD is beginning to seriously impact their physical health and mental wellbeing (e.g. refusing food and drink, leading to malnutrition and dehydration), which may necessitate an involuntary hospital stay for life-saving treatment. The person is said to be 'sectioned', a term referring to one of the sections of the Mental Health Act.

Mental Capacity Act 2005

The Mental Capacity Act is another key piece of government legislation to support those lacking capacity to make important decisions. The principles of the Act state that a person is assumed to have capacity unless it is established that they lack capacity. To demonstrate capacity, the individual must be able to understand and retain information, show they are able to debate the pros and cons of any decision, and communicate their decision clearly verbally or in writing. Decisions about capacity are time- and situation-specific. Capacity may relate to decisions about the person's health, but also other related aspects, such as financial and legal decisions.

Unlike the Mental Health Act, the Mental Capacity Act recognises that a person's capacity can be temporary or fluctuate over time – for example, due to a head injury, pain, or the effects of drugs or alcohol. It is also important to remember that individuals may have the capacity to make decisions that professionals or family members consider unwise. Such decisions can sometimes lead to distress or tension among relatives and healthcare staff. We see this clinically manifest in maternity settings, where a patient may be advised by staff to have a medically assisted birth/caesarean section, but the parent is reluctant, insisting on a 'natural', unassisted birth. In cases where the severity puts life in danger, an urgent Court of Protection Order may be requested for support surrounding obstetric decision-making. In such complex presentations, it would be imperative to state whether a mental health diagnosis is impacting on their ability to decide about their care.

Deprivations of liberty

Deprivations of Liberty Safeguards (DoLs) may be necessary when a person cannot make decisions for themselves, such as when hospital treatment or admission to a care home is needed. Included within the Mental Capacity Act, DoLs provide a legal framework to protect individuals' rights by ensuring that they are only deprived of liberty when it is in their best interests and using the least restrictive option. UK health professionals must submit applications to the local authority or Court of Protection and conduct regular assessments of DoLs, following protocols to ensure safeguarding measures are appropriate, reasonable, and based on the latest risk assessments.

SAFEGUARDING

Safeguarding vulnerable women, children, and families is central to perinatal mental health practice, as well as all services involved in caring for these groups. Hospitals, schools, and places of worship typically have safeguarding policies and often designate a safeguarding lead or guardian. This person can provide advice and support and advocate for the appropriate pathways in the best interests of the individual (Department of Health 1998).

It is essential for health professionals to always uphold a duty of care with the best interests of both the child and the mother. On rare occasions, this may require consultation with multiple agencies to support and protect those in need. However, understanding perinatal mental health, particularly perinatal OCD, is vital to ensuring fair and suitable care pathways are established.

It is crucial for health professionals to consistently uphold a duty of care that prioritises the best interests of both the child and the mother. In rare cases, this may involve consulting multiple agencies to support and safeguard those in need. Nevertheless, understanding perinatal mental health, especially perinatal OCD, is essential to ensuring that fair and appropriate care pathways are in place. Correctly diagnosing perinatal OCD is vital. It helps prevent staff from mistakenly viewing disclosed obsessional fears as risk, which could lead to unnecessary social service referrals and traumatic experiences for patients. Accurate understanding ensures safe, appropriate support, avoiding harmful decisions.

In the next chapter, I specify how to accurately assess and diagnose perinatal OCD to avoid such tragic misunderstandings in clinical practice.

CHAPTER 12

Classification and Assessment of Perinatal OCD

As discussed in the previous chapter, an inaccurate diagnosis can have devastating consequences for the patient and the family, with potential to lead down a path to further assessment under the Mental Health Act or where safeguarding concerns may be raised. In this chapter, I provide an overview of assessing perinatal OCD using formal classification, screening tools, and clinical assessment.

CLASSIFICATION

To make an accurate diagnosis of OCD (and to differentiate from other types of mental illnesses), health professionals are not only reliant on their clinical acumen but must make a diagnosis in keeping with the *International Classification of Diseases* (ICD) manual in the UK and Europe; the equivalent in the US is the *Diagnostic and Statistical Manual* (DSM). The ICD is reviewed regularly by experts in the field. The updated 11th edition includes several subtle but relevant changes to OCD spectrum related disorders. For example, hoarding and body dysmorphic disorder are recognised as their own unique clinical conditions, which I discuss more in Chapter 13. Mental and behavioural disorders come under one of the chapters of the ICD-11, with OCD a specific subcategory of neurotic, stress-related, and somatoform disorders.

PERINATAL OCD: HIDDEN IN BROAD DAYLIGHT

Perinatal OCD often remains hidden because patients do not report symptoms, and clinicians may not detect it. Although some women experience both postnatal OCD and postnatal depression, postnatal OCD is mostly clinically distinct from depression, sharing more features with postnatal anxiety.

Perinatal OCD is marked by an overwhelming worry that does not settle with reassurance. Although some patients can hide their symptoms, by the time the baby arrives, the worries are often shared with family members, who do their best to reassure and even at times support the compulsive behaviours. This can temporarily reduce the mother's anxieties, putting her and everyone else at ease. By the time it reaches the attention of a GP or health professional, the patient and their family have been learning to live with it for months, or even years, making adaptations to their daily routines to accommodate the obsessions and compulsions. For example, partners and parents may:

- offer constant reassurance
- help with obsessional rituals, such as checking the bath temperature
- limit social outings
- feed the baby a certain way
- avoid triggering situations (such as withholding reassurance or not agreeing to partake in checking behaviours).

The condition is characterised by a lot of activity, as it requires significant energy both to ruminate on worries and to perform compulsions. In contrast, postnatal depression is marked by a lack of ability to maintain normal energy levels (Dorfan & Woody 2012). Patients with postnatal depression present quite differently in clinic compared to those with postnatal OCD. They may appear lethargic, with a flat mood, reduced eye contact, and tears during the assessment. Conversely, patients with postnatal OCD may seem quite well, until you start discussing their thoughts, at which point even talking about them may fill them with dread and show visible signs of anxiety (Burton 2021).

During assessment for OCD, one must also be aware of the increased likelihood of co-existing conditions that would need assessment and/or treatment. Patients presenting with OCD may have an increased risk of clinical depression and anxiety, as well as substance misuse. They may also present to other services, such as dermatology clinics, where their OCD or body dysmorphia may manifest through concerns about their skin or appearance. Other common conditions alongside OCD include movement disorders, such as tics and Tourette syndrome.

SAMPLE ASSESSMENT QUESTIONS FOR OCD AND PERINATAL OCD

These sample questions are by no means an exhaustive list but provide a guide to conversation points in clinical practice to allow for more in-depth information sharing. Be mindful that for many women with pre-existing or new-onset symptoms this might be the first time they have been asked personal questions about their thoughts and rituals in such detail. Note the importance of time spent engaging in the behaviours and whether the behaviour/compulsions negatively affect the patient, both of which will allow the clinician to form an impression about how these symptoms are affecting quality of life and activities of daily living.

- Do you wash or clean a lot?
- Do you check things a lot?
- Is there any thought that keeps bothering you that you would like to get rid of but can't?
- Do your daily activities take a long time to finish?
- Are you concerned about putting things in a special order or are you very upset by mess?
- Do these problems trouble you?

Pregnancy-specific questions

For a patient who is pregnant, you may want to consider asking additional questions such as:

- Do you have any particular worries about the health of the unborn child?
- Do you find yourself wanting to check on the baby more often, with an urge to book extra scan appointments?

- Do you have any concerns about the paternity of the unborn child?
- Have you made any significant changes to your diet and/or lifestyle in relation to your pregnancy (limiting certain foods, avoiding certain places or people, avoiding public transport, etc.)?
- Do you find yourself 'google-searching' about statistics around miscarriages and/or pregnancy/birth complications?
- If you have experienced OCD in the past, do you feel that it has got worse during pregnancy? If so, in what way?
- Did you take medication for your mental health previously and/or stop medication when you found out you were pregnant?

Postnatal-specific questions

Sample questions that can be useful after the baby has been born include:

- Are you bottle feeding, breastfeeding, or a combination of both? Did any intrusive thoughts or worries influence your choice of feeding method?
- Do you have any concerns around your breast milk, or the act of breastfeeding?
- Are you worried that you may pass on any illness or disease through your breast milk, or through touching/close contact?
- Do you get any unwanted sexual thoughts whilst breastfeeding, or have you had any worries that people may think you are a paedophile when you are feeding or looking after your baby?
- Do you have any worries about harm coming to your baby?
- Do you find yourself checking on your baby through the night?
- Do usual baby routines (feeding/bath time) take a long time?
- Do you have a specific set of routines for yourself and the children, when doing certain tasks or leaving the house?
- If you get interrupted or make a mistake, do you feel compelled to start the routines all over again?
- Have you booked a lot of appointments with specialists/health professionals? Or are you attending urgent care centres because of concerns about your child ?

- Do you find yourself repeatedly sterilising baby bottles/cleaning the house/washing baby linen and clothes? And (if yes) despite doing all of this, does it never feel 'clean enough'?
- Have you avoided having visitors, letting people touch the baby, going out to certain places such as appointments or baby groups, or using public transport (for fear of contamination/harm)?
- Have you experienced any unwanted intrusive visual images of significant harm coming to your child ('flash-forward' of a worst-case scenario, such as an image of baby covered in blood or a fatal accident)?

SCREENING TOOLS

Screening tools are often used in clinical practice. Usually in the form of a short questionnaire, they provide additional information to support making a diagnosis. There are a range of screening tools used in primary care and perinatal mental health services, such as the Edinburgh Postnatal Depression Scale and the Generalised Anxiety Disorder Questionnaire. In maternity services, the Whooley Questionnaire is a two-question screening tool for depression asked at every booking appointment nationwide.

The Yale-Brown Obsessive Compulsive Scale (Y-BOCS) is the gold standard objective screening tool used by clinicians. It includes a comprehensive, detailed symptom checklist of current and past symptoms, as well as a scale to assess time spent on OCD, the distress it causes, and other important features such as avoidance, impact on relationships, insight, and perceived feelings surrounding responsibility and doubt.

The scale can be used for children and adults but must be administered and scored by a clinician. There is a growing trend towards self-administered screening tools, such as the Obsessive-Compulsive Inventory (OCI). These do not require specialist training and can be completed by the patient themselves. Although it has 42 questions, it balances being detailed enough with being quick and easy to complete, making it suitable for use in community mental health and maternity settings.

To date, there are no specific screening tools for perinatal OCD available for use in clinical practice. The questionnaires available do not explore in detail the nuances of perinatal OCD, and scoring may be unreliable as they do not account for thoughts about harm to the baby. To make an accurate diagnosis of perinatal OCD, clinicians must rely on careful history-taking and assessment.

CHAPTER 13

Differential Diagnoses

As important as it is to know and understand what perinatal OCD is, we also need to understand what it isn't. One challenge with this complex condition is that it is often confused with other diagnoses. This is understandable as many of the common symptoms overlap. In this chapter, I discuss conditions which are mistakenly diagnosed when working with women with OCD, delineating their key features to show how they differ from perinatal OCD.

Although traditionally in scientific disciplines we gravitate towards categorisation and classification, life is rarely that linear and diagnoses rarely that distinct in clinical practice. It is very possible for patients to experience more than one condition at the same time (e.g. both perinatal OCD and depression, or perinatal OCD and body dysmorphia). This can pose further challenges for the focus of treatment. However, the perinatal OCD aspect is relatively easy to identify, if the treating clinician understands the condition and the condition is detected in a timely manner (Fornaro et al. 2009).

What are the odds?

About one in four women will face a clinical mental health challenge – such as anxiety, depression, or OCD – either during pregnancy or in the year after childbirth. Fortunately, postnatal psychosis is quite rare, affecting about 1 in 1000 women, but it's a serious condition that can develop suddenly within days of delivery, even in women with no previous psychiatric history. Although a rare condition, the risk level is similar to that of a mother under 35 having a baby with Down syndrome. Think about how much education, advice, and conversations happen about Down syndrome during antenatal care. Sadly, the conversations and awareness about postnatal psychosis and other perinatal mental health conditions during pregnancy remain very limited and often silent, which is something we need to change.

POSTNATAL DEPRESSION

Postnatal depression is arguably the most common condition in the perinatal period. Approximately one in five mothers experience this illness after the birth of their child. Depressive features can occur any time during the perinatal period. Those presenting in the postnatal period were likely experiencing symptoms of depression during pregnancy, which, coincidentally, is just as common, affecting one in five women. These facts go against the expectations placed upon expectant mothers to be happy, lucky, and grateful at all times.

The realities of pregnancy, labour, and the postpartum period are often glossed over, minimising the multitude of complex factors that can affect the mother, her pregnancy, and her relationship with the baby. Factors affecting one's mood include, but are not limited to:

- previous experiences of baby loss, including miscarriage, stillbirth, neonatal death, removal of children by social care or adoption
- obstetric complications in pregnancy affecting the mother
- severe pregnancy symptoms, including morning sickness, poor appetite, pelvic pain, and symphysis pubis disorder
- pre-existing medical conditions that need to be managed/monitored in pregnancy
- medication adherence in pregnancy and breastfeeding (worry whether it may harm the unborn)
- foetal complications, including growth and developmental abnormalities

- circumstances leading to conception and relationship dynamics with the father of the child
- mother's understanding of motherhood, and her experience of parenting/being parented
- financial challenges
- conflicts over maternity leave and return to work
- fear of childbirth (tokophobia)
- traumatic birth experience
- difficulties in establishing breastfeeding
- guilt, pressure, or negative feelings surrounding infant feeding choices
- neonatal conditions requiring hospitalisation and additional care (e.g. neonatal jaundice, neonatal surgery, or tongue tie).

Some believe that postnatal depression is 'just regular depression occurring in the postnatal period'. This is true to a certain extent. As outlined in the ICD-11, the core symptoms of depression remain the same, with no special caveats for those in the perinatal period:

- anhedonia (loss of pleasure)
- reduced energy
- low mood
- biological symptoms such as poor sleep, appetite, and libido.

After giving birth, all new mothers, regardless of having additional family support, feel tired and experience reduced energy, poor sleep, and reduced sexual drive, ticking the list of the ICD-11 classification for symptoms of a depressive episode.

One must be mindful of this when assessing women and pay close attention to the nature and duration of the symptoms. If feelings of low mood persist for longer than two weeks and/or there is a history of depression (either during pregnancy or in their medical background), then postnatal depression should be considered a strong possibility, and treatment should be offered promptly, as it can deteriorate rapidly, putting both mother and baby at risk. If postnatal depression remains untreated, it can worsen considerably. The mother may experience features of psychosis, mainly preoccupied with guilt and feeling worthless as a mother. These feelings could be accompanied by thoughts of harming herself or the baby, believing they would be 'better off' without them. I discuss this in more detail in the postnatal psychosis subsection below.

'Just a bit of baby blues'

Baby blues is a specific yet common hormonal rebalancing phenomenon, affecting as much as 75% of new mothers whether they have experienced mental health issues before or not. This rebalancing typically peaks at three to five days post-delivery, the condition resolves spontaneously without intervention within a week of giving birth. Symptoms include:

- feelings of underwhelm
- irritability
- crying more than usual.

I have met countless women, referred just before their child's first birthday, who have been depressed pretty much the whole year. When questioned, they note having had symptoms since delivery that continued through the year. Friends, family, and even health professionals told them not to worry as it was 'just a bit of baby blues'.

Postnatal depression verses postnatal OCD[1]

When trying to determine whether it is postnatal depression or postnatal OCD that a mother is experiencing, consider the key differences of each as described above. However, remember that the most appropriate action is to refer the patient to a specialist perinatal mental health service for a formal assessment and diagnosis. No one expects time-pressured frontline staff in primary care, maternity, or community services to diagnose mental health disorders. Instead, they should be aware of the signs and know when to refer patients to specialist services.

1 As mentioned in Chapter 1, 'perinatal OCD' and 'postnatal OCD' are often used interchangeably. In this context, I use postnatal OCD as a comparison with postnatal depression, for symptoms of OCD emerging after delivery – either as new onset or a relapse of a pre-existing OCD.

In postnatal OCD, anxiety is the primary 'family' of issues that the condition arises from. It overlaps with both depression and general anxiety, with many patients experiencing all three. However, with depression, the symptoms are mainly centred around a persistent low mood that is hard to shift. During moderate to severe episodes of clinical depression, one cannot simply 'snap out of it' by meeting friends, reading a book, or doing some exercise. Although these activities may provide temporary relief, they are not a cure.

Those experiencing depression may describe feeling a 'black cloud' over them, where basic tasks and daily activities feel like a huge chore. With 'high-functioning' depression or anxiety, some can continue to work and fulfil their various roles and family commitments, keeping all the plates spinning, but when left alone, they feel very worn down and depressed. In fact, for these women, the demands of career and family life on their time become a welcome distraction. When facing maternity leave, alone with their baby and without the buffers of a busy work schedule, symptoms of depression can surface.

POSTNATAL ANXIETY

Anxiety can be described as an 'umbrella' term. In anxiety, several different disorders co-exist, either separately or sometimes grouped together. OCD is one of the conditions that exist under the broader category of anxiety disorders. Other related conditions include:

- simple phobias
- panic attacks
- generalised anxiety disorder
- social anxiety
- claustrophobia
- agoraphobia.

Collectively, these are the most prevalent mental health conditions worldwide, carrying the highest economic costs. Although each condition above has its own specific symptoms, they all share the core theme of worry, usually about a specific thing, person, or place. Anxiety disorders often produce a physical manifestation with visible clinical symptoms of stress, including:

- increased heart rate
- changes to breathing
- feeling startled
- dizziness
- sweating
- palpitations
- in the case of a panic attack, a 'fear of impending doom' where one feels they might die, thus experiencing an overwhelming need to escape the situation by any means possible.

Mindful and meditative initiatives can be helpful, to an extent. However, in acute anxiety or panic attacks where the fear is at its most severe, simply telling someone to relax rarely works, as the fear cannot be controlled or directed.

For the mothers attending my clinic, I often state something quite controversial – that motherhood itself is anxiety-provoking, and that it would be quite unusual (and possibly pathological) if mothers weren't anxious about anything at all, particularly their baby's wellbeing. One may experience other related anxiety disorders co-occurring with perinatal OCD (given its prevalence of approximately 1 in 5 women experiencing clinical anxiety during their lifetime).

In a 'simple' anxiety disorder, worries may be widespread and often catastrophised, but they tend to persist with the individual, leading to continuous rumination without specific compulsive actions to stop it. The main sign that differentiates OCD is anxiety driven by obsessional, intrusive, and distressing thoughts, along with attempts to 'neutralise' the underlying fear through compulsive behaviours, routines, and rituals. As noted earlier, these behaviours can be creative and vary from mental repetitions to avoidance or physical manifestations. Some research indicates that individuals who develop OCD in later life or during the perinatal period may have had anxiety disorders during childhood (Brandes, Soares, & Cohen 2004).

Tokophobia: Fear of childbirth

Because tokophobia is a condition that many health professionals encounter with expectant mothers, it is important to both understand and manage it appropriately. Tokophobia is a mental health condition characterised by an intense fear of pregnancy or childbirth. Anxiety about the 'unknowns' of pregnancy and labour is common and somewhat expected, especially for first-time mothers. It can manifest as a severe clinical condition that not only influences a woman's feelings about labour but also affects how she might choose to give birth, often opting for an elective caesarean section, sometimes under general anaesthetic.

Factors that can influence or trigger tokophobia include:

- past traumatic birth experiences (including infant loss)
- stories from other women about negative birth experiences
- past traumatic events, including sexual abuse, assault, or rape
- pre-existing anxiety disorder (now with a new focus of the pregnancy)
- fear of practical aspects of the maternity care (including fear of hospitals or fear of needles)
- a history of gynaecological conditions that may lead to a more complicated, high-risk pregnancy, triggering anxiety.

Aspects of necessary care may be affected and thus avoided, including:

- internal (vaginal) examinations
- ultrasound scans (particularly in early pregnancy as it is often internally performed transvaginally)
- induction of labour and of pain relief.

Severe tokophobia not only affects the mother's care but also impacts the unborn child. Fear of pregnancy and childbirth may lead to refusal or avoidance of monitoring the baby's development *in utero*, including screening tests, scans, and procedures that might be necessary during delivery. Conversely, some patients may seek repeated reassurance through additional antenatal scans and investigations and may strongly prefer a caesarean section to avoid the pain of childbirth.

Health anxiety

Health anxiety is an increasingly common presentation, particularly in recent years with public health concerns and governance around COVID-19 and the vaccination programme. Presentations can be broadly divided into two categories: those who have anxiety about medical symptoms, such as bloating, dizziness, or headache (sometimes referred to as somatoform disorder) and those who are worried they may have a serious medical condition, such as cancer (previously called hypochondriasis).

In clinical practice, it can be challenging to distinguish between health anxiety and OCD presentations, as both involve a common pattern of anxiety with reassurance-seeking, particularly from health professionals. Many patients frequently visit hospitals or outpatient clinics, request multiple medical investigations, or engage in 'doctor shopping', trying to find a cause for their unexplained symptoms. The patient may obsessively google their perceived symptoms or review online chat forums, sacrificing their sleep and wellbeing in the process.

Some patients may experience a severe form of health anxiety called hypochondriasis. This condition falls within the obsessive-compulsive spectrum and is characterised by a persistent preoccupation with the fear of having one or more serious or life-threatening diseases. Although they may fear death or dying, in OCD they recognise this as untrue and often remark that they know their thoughts are 'ridiculous'. The patient with health anxiety or hypochondriasis, however, is less certain about this. They often appear highly anxious, convinced they have a medical issue that has been missed. Making an accurate diagnosis requires patience and careful collaboration with the GP and specialists. Those who frequently attend emergency services may need additional support and discussions with A&E staff to develop a care plan aimed at reducing unnecessary crisis visits.

Factitious disorder imposed upon another (FDIOA)

The 2021 novel *Darling Rose Gold* by Staphanie Wrobel is a chilling psychological thriller about the twisted relationship between a mother and daughter. The novel captured the public fascination with Munchausen's syndrome by proxy, recounting the story of a mother imprisoned for 18 years after being found guilty of fabricating and inducing illness in her child. The illness, first described in 1977, has had several names including factitious disorder, fabricated and induced illness in children (FII), factitious disorder imposed on another (FDIOA), or, more recently in the US, medical child abuse. These name variations reflect the confusions and tensions within the relationships between those involved, whether as children, caregivers, and professionals or victims, perpetrators, and enablers. In the UK, the condition is formally referred to as FDIOA, though many people are familiar with the older terminology of Munchausen's syndrome by proxy. The research surrounding FDIOA acknowledges that the condition exists as a spectrum of healthcare-seeking behaviour in the parent (usually the mother) and that either extreme can put the child at risk. Behaviours range from not seeking care for the child (extreme neglect) to that of over-seeking care and fabricating illness.

To date, there are no research studies specifically examining the crossover between perinatal OCD and FDIOA. However, both theoretically and clinically, we may observe evidence of blurred lines involving increased health-seeking behaviour and abnormal illness behaviour, alongside comorbidities such as health anxiety, depression, Asperger's syndrome, and somatoform disorders. The key difference in FDIOA, however, is that the caregiver (usually the mother) consciously and deliberately provides false information about the child's welfare to elicit the desired response from health professionals. The patient may exaggerate symptoms, fabricate stories about the child's history, or misinterpret real-life events due to mistaken beliefs about their significance. Physical deception may also occur through tampering with medical records, interfering with investigations and specimens, or, in extreme cases, inducing signs of illness in the child through poisoning or overuse of medication. Presentations can vary from concerns about the child having an actual illness or allergy to reports that the child exhibits behavioural issues or is not developing normally. Children may be presented as unable to walk, not toilet trained, or unable to eat normal food. The presentation is particularly concerning if detected during the perinatal period, as the child cannot advocate for themselves (Bass & Glaser 2014).

Regarding the assessment and management of such presentations, the cases may be extremely complex and often involve several different health professionals from various specialties and even different locations, as the perpetrator may 'shop around' seeking validation and/or a diagnosis. Although the requests may appear obsessive, they lack the typical ego-dystonic fear associated with OCD. Health professionals must also report any concerns to children and family safeguarding and child protection pathways. Such cases can lead to serious incidents that may require investigation, and health professionals might be required to present evidence in court (Royal College of Psychiatrists 2020).

BODY DYSMORPHIC DISORDER

Body dysmorphia is characterised by an intense focus on a specific body part or aspect of one's appearance. It can also manifest as a general dislike and discomfort with one's body, feeling that it is 'not quite right' and needs to be altered before they, or others, can accept it. The condition was previously classified as a subset of OCD because of similar obsessive traits. The key in making a differential diagnosis is that in OCD the intrusive thoughts and repetitive behaviours are not limited solely to physical appearance as they are in body dysmorphic disorder (Phillips & Kelly 2021).

Research into body dysmorphia has progressed significantly over the past decade, possibly due to the increase in cases linked to the image-conscious sphere of social media, promotion of filters, and Photoshop technologies affecting self-perception (Laughter et al. 2023). As understanding of the condition has improved, we are beginning to see a subtle but clear shift away from considering it a subset of OCD to recognising it as a standalone condition on the spectrum, sometimes involving fixed and paranoid beliefs. This is reflected in treatment approaches, where targeted treatments aimed at delusional thinking appear to be beneficial in those body dysmorphia, such as antipsychotics (Rossell et al. 2020). However, specialists remain divided about labelling the condition as delusional in nature, preferring to refer to it as an 'overvalued idea', which may be concurrent with OCD particularly in adolescence (Conceição Costa et al. 2012; de Leon, Bott, & Simpson 1989).

In practice, patients with body dysmorphia are more likely to present to outpatient surgical clinics than to psychiatry clinics, as they seek practical solutions through cosmetic procedures to alter their physical appearance. A notable feature of this condition is the request for repeated surgical, dental, or dermatological interventions (often shopping around or paying privately to reduce the risk of being denied services), coupled with decreased satisfaction scores observed after surgery.

Body dysmorphia in pregnancy and the postnatal period

As we mentioned in the introduction to Part 2, matrescence is a period of biological, physical, hormonal, and psychological changes for a woman transitioning to motherhood. It is common for women to experience mixed emotions about the body changes during pregnancy or in the postnatal period. Significant alterations in the size and shape of a woman's body during and after pregnancy constitute a unique form of body dysmorphia common in the perinatal period. Physical changes that occur during pregnancy that could become a focus include but are not limited to:

- the size and shape of the abdomen and widening of hips
- changes to the size, colour, and shape of breasts and/or nipples, or preoccupation with lactation (concerns about the quantity and/or quality of the breast milk)
- weight gain and struggling to fit into one's pre-pregnancy clothes
- postpartum hair loss (telogen effluvium) caused by fluctuating hormone levels, specifically a reduction in oestrogen, which peaks two to four months postnatal
- swollen legs and increase in size of feet

- skin changes, such as developing the linea nigra (a vertical darker line on the surface of the belly) or appearance of stretch marks
- vaginal changes, particularly if one experiences trauma during childbirth, such as a vaginal tear, or functional difficulties such as urinary incontinence.

Although diagnosing body dysmorphic disorder is challenging in this subgroup, it's crucial to consider OCD and BDD if the patient's concerns seem disproportionate to typical perinatal experiences. Clinicians should be mindful of and empathetic towards women's bodily experiences during the perinatal period, which may be intensified by societal obsession with appearance, high beauty standards, and the postnatal 'snapback culture'.

EATING DISORDERS

The link between eating disorders and OCD has been recognised for some time. A study by Kaye et al. (2004) estimates that 10% of people with OCD will experience an eating disorder at some point in their lives. Both anorexia nervosa and OCD share common cognitive, biological, and personality traits, particularly perfectionism, heightened anxiety, and emotional dysregulation when they cannot exert control over their fears. Some also argue that both conditions involve the same neurobiological circuitry and that the very nature of eating disorders can mirror the pattern of OCD; the core 'fear of fatness' leads to repetitive and persistent obsessional beliefs about body image and a desire to lose weight, countered by ritualised eating patterns and over-exercising (Ortiz et al. 2022).

Both OCD and eating disorders can cause serious medical complications. People with eating disorders often restrict their diet, leading to deficiencies such as anaemia, osteopenia, metabolic acidosis, bradycardia, dehydration, and hyponatraemia. OCD can also result in restrictive eating or drinking, which may affect renal function, although the underlying fear might not be of fatness itself but rather contamination (Flamarique et al. 2019).

The key difference between the two conditions, however, is whether the primary fears and obsessional thoughts are ego-dystonic or ego-syntonic. In OCD, they are ego-dystonic; people are repulsed and embarrassed by their core fears. In eating disorders, they are ego-syntonic; people are wedded to the pursuit of thinness. Some have argued that eating disorders are not an obsessional fear but an overvalued idea possibly with delusional intensity (Barton et al. 2022).

It was believed for many years that women with severe eating disorders did not reach the perinatal stage. This belief stemmed from the misconception that severe anorexia nervosa would stop their periods and hinder their ability to conceive. Nowadays, we are seeing an increase in women with past and present eating disorders becoming pregnant, and these women benefit from multidisciplinary expert-led care due to the complexity of their condition and the potential impact that restrictive eating can have on the developing foetus.

Body image in the perinatal period

Many women struggle with natural and expected body changes during the perinatal period, as reflected in our societal obsession with 'snapping back' to our pre-pregnancy bodies and weight. As Susie Orbach discusses in her governmental guidance *Two for the Price of One* (Orbach & Rubin 2014), body-image difficulties often manifest in pregnancy. If not addressed, they can impact the longer-term bond and attachment with the baby, as the mother is subconsciously preoccupied with 'erasing' the evidence of her pregnancy and fixated on fitting into her 'pre-pregnancy jeans'.

Body-image issues are inherently linked with disordered eating and eating disorders (two distinct entities). They can be passed on through the generations, reinforced by cultural and societal expectations. Although eating disorders in the perinatal period are outside the realm of this book, be aware of the overlapping themes of overvalued ideas surrounding body image, weight, and ruminations on food and exercise, particularly in the postnatal period. This is something that may require further assessment and/or intervention.

Whether the diagnosis of an eating disorder or OCD is present, we know that both exist on a spectrum involving obsessive-compulsive symptoms, body-image concerns, and society's obsession with the 'snapback' body postpartum. It may be that prior to pregnancy, the mother (even without the label of an eating disorder) skilfully managed her weight through a careful balance of a strict diet and regular exercise, a behaviour she may have engaged in from a young age. Once pregnant, the diet is disrupted (in fact, for most women, it is advised not to diet but to add an additional 500 calories per day). They may also vomit more frequently or have specific food cravings or aversions, which may trigger emetophobia (fear of vomiting) and OCD.

Orthorexia nervosa

In the last decade, we have seen a sharp rise in the 'clean eating' movement, with a fixation not only on the quantity of food eaten, but the quality. Orthorexia nervosa can be defined as pathological fixation or obsession with proper nutrition, characterised by a restrictive diet, ritualised patterns of eating, and rigid avoidance of foods believed to be unhealthy or impure. Although prompted by a desire to achieve optimum health, orthorexia may lead to nutritional deficiencies, medical complications, and poor quality of life (Yilmaz et al. 2020).

Although the condition was first described in the late 1990s by physician Steven Bratman, it is yet to be officially included in the ICD or DSM, as the debate continues over whether orthorexia nervosa should be recognised as a diagnosable medical condition. Characteristics include:

- obsessional preoccupation on the 'purity' of foods
- excessive scrutiny on the source of foods (e.g. exposure to pesticides, processing, micro-nutrients, addition of artificial flavourings and preservatives)

- packaging concerns (whether food may contain plastic-derived and/or carcinogenic compounds).

For those living with orthorexia nervosa, there is often an element of dietary restriction. They may exclude food groups such as processed and 'junk' foods, meat, dairy, grains, and non-seasonal, non-organic fruits and vegetables. Not only is this practice costly in terms of financial commitment, but also of time taken with obsessional and compulsive behaviours. Similar to social avoidant behaviour in OCD, people with orthorexia nervosa often avoid socialising and eating with others as they may not share the same belief systems as them around food (Koven & Abry 2015).

A handful of studies to date have examined the relationship between OCD and orthorexia nervosa (e.g. Cosh, Olson, & Tully 2023; Zagaria et al. 2022). Although most study participants were women of childbearing age, no pregnant or postnatal women were included. From our own clinical experience on the front line of perinatal mental health services, we know that there is increased attention to detail regarding diet during pregnancy and breastfeeding. While partly driven by concerns about certain food consumption and its risks to the baby, it is also related to a maternal desire to consume high-quality food to pass on 'the best' nutrients to the unborn, which may sometimes display some orthorexia nervosa tendencies. This could be an extension of a pre-existing eating disorder/orthorexia nervosa or a new phenomenon and desire to be as healthy as possible in the perinatal period. The desire for pure, organic food may persist into the postnatal period, especially around weaning, with careful attention and time spent preparing organic homemade purees to feed the baby (Pontillo et al. 2022).

HOARDING DISORDER

When I was Psychiatry Senior Registrar, I will never forget my first encounter with severe hoarding during a home visit assessment. I was called to a townhouse in a quiet London suburb to join the mental health assessment team. Getting through the front door was a struggle as I had to climb over piles of old newspapers stacked so high they reached my shoulders. Inside, the kitchen was filled with books, newspapers, and magazines from floor to ceiling. A gas hob was hidden amongst the junk, indicating a clear fire hazard. On meeting the elderly woman on the top floor, she appeared malnourished and unwell. She described herself as a 'collector' and appeared unaware of the concerns her daughter and the mental health team had about her wellbeing. After assessing the risks, the team unanimously decided she needed hospital care.

Hoarding and OCD have historically been linked, often caused by the misconception that OCD equates to an obsession with tidying and organisation. While these conditions share some similarities, hoarding disorder is now acknowledged as a separate clinical diagnosis within the spectrum of OCD and related disorders.

In hoarding disorder, a person exhibits a significant accumulation of possessions, either because they buy or collect many items or have difficulty discarding them (often both). Items may be valuable but are usually considered trash by most, such as old magazines or empty bottles. The behaviour of accumulation is like the compulsive aspect of OCD and is driven by repetitive, obsessive urges to acquire more, as well as anxiety around discarding items. Levels of self-awareness vary but are usually compromised when anxiety is high. Over time, living spaces become so cluttered that they are uninhabitable and may pose serious environmental risks, as well as interfering with personal hygiene, family relationships, and daily functioning (OCD-UK 2025a).

Although it is a relatively uncommon presentation during pregnancy and postnatal, it is something to consider, particularly in those that may be experiencing depression, anxiety, OCD, or grief reaction. As with all mental health conditions in the perinatal period, one must always be mindful of the risks posed to the baby, and whether the circumstances warrant referral to children and family social care/safeguarding processes. Through standard home visits by various health professionals during the perinatal period (such as health visitors, midwives, and mental health nurses), hoarding disorder has the potential to be detected, and thus treated, much earlier compared with the non-pregnant hoarding population.

Alongside hoarding, there are other conditions that are recognised as related disorders to OCD. In Table 13.1, I have summarised a collection of conditions related to OCD that one may encounter in clinical practice alongside OCD in the perinatal period.

Table 13.1. OCD-related disorders

Disorder	Description
Tics, including both physical and vocal tics	Physical tics are fast repetitive muscle movements that cause sudden bodily movement, jolts, or noises that are difficult to control. They include: • blinking • eye rolling • grimacing • shoulder shrugging • jerking of the head or limbs • jumping • twirling • touching objects and other people. Vocal tics include: • grunting • throat clearing • whistling • coughing • tongue clicking • animal sounds • saying random words and phrases • repeating a sound, word, or phrase • swearing.
Tourette syndrome	Combination of physical and vocal tics. Common condition in childhood but can also be associated with ADHD, ASD, and anxiety disorder.
Dermatillomania (also known as excoriation disorder or skin-picking disorder)	The compulsion to pick at one's own skin, freckles, pimples, moles, spots, or scars. May have the urge to 'smooth' out areas of imperfection. Includes picking, rubbing, pinching, squeezing, or biting and can increase in times of heightened stress and anxiety.
Trichotillomania (hair-pulling disorder)	The urge/compulsion to pull one's own hair (from their scalp, eyebrows, eyelashes, body hair, armpit, or genital area).

AUTISM SPECTRUM DISORDER

Autism spectrum disorder (ASD) is a neurodevelopmental condition characterised by challenges in social communication, repetitive behaviours, and restricted repertoire of interests.

ASD shares many similarities with OCD. In clinical practice, the two are often confused with one another (Postorino et al. 2017). Common symptoms include:

- intrusive recurrent thoughts
- repetitive compulsive-like behaviours
- following strict rituals and routines with marked distress if unable to adhere to these (often self-imposed) rules.

Individuals with OCD and/or ASD uniquely have insight into their thoughts. Although in some cases, their thinking may appear rigid or fixed to a certain degree, they are not considered delusional. Key differences between OCD and autism are found in the details. Those on the autism spectrum are often very sensitive to sensory stimuli and may engage in repetitive acts because they find the act to be soothing and somewhat comforting (e.g. stroking a jumper because they like the soft feel of the yarn, or flicking the light switches on and off because they enjoy the 'clicking' sound it makes and the visual stimulus of the lamp illuminating).

In OCD, compulsive behaviours are something that 'must' be done to stop harm or a bad thing from happening (e.g. switching the gas hob on and off 20 times means that the hob is working and there will not be a gas leak or house fire).

The traditional view that ASD is a 'male-only' condition has evolved in recent years. Women and girls are increasingly recognised as autistic as much as men and boys. In clinical practice, we are witnessing an emerging phenomenon of women who may be autistic, where a diagnosis was missed in childhood and is now manifesting during the perinatal period. Women on the autism spectrum often find the increasing demands of pregnancy and the postnatal period challenging. This may be for several reasons, including:

- high societal expectations and pressures placed on pregnant women and new mothers coupled with perfectionist desires
- relative lack of control (to changing body, the labour process, and having a newborn)
- changes to routine
- reduced ability to stick to preferred rituals once baby arrives

- increased sensory overwhelm (from foetal movements in pregnancy to baby crying in the postnatal period)
- increased expectation for medical examinations and social interactions with health professionals, friends, and family through the perinatal period.
- struggles with bonding and attachment in the postnatal period, due to difficulties in reading facial and social cues and managing the intimate relationship with a newborn whose main way of communicating their needs is through crying.

Of course, someone can be autistic and also experience perinatal OCD. Staff working with women during the perinatal period need to have increased understanding and awareness of autism in women to be able to detect the condition as well as specific training on how to support those with neurodivergence during pregnancy and postpartum.

SCHIZOPHRENIA AND RELATED DISORDERS

Schizophrenia is a complex and serious mental illness characterised by a person's detachment from reality, namely through a combination of delusional beliefs (a fixed, false, and unshakeable belief that is not in keeping with cultural and societal values) and abnormal sensory experiences commonly known as hallucinations. Dr Emile Kraepelin first identified it as a distinguishable psychiatric disorder in 1887. Since then, our knowledge of the condition has grown considerably. Schizophrenia, like many other mental health difficulties, manifests on a spectrum of psychosis-related disorders, including:

- schizo-affective disorder
- persistent paranoid disorder
- various forms of psychosis, such as drug-induced, stress-induced, and postnatal (puerperal) psychosis.

Rarely, women may experience delusions of pregnancy or pseudocyesis (phantom pregnancy) – a condition where one is convinced they are pregnant with objective pregnancy signs in the absence of a positive pregnancy test. The fixation on pregnancy may be mistaken for obsession, particularly as the thoughts are often recurring and all-consuming, taking up a lot of time and energy for both the patient and all staff involved. These patients may also have other mental health issues, not just psychosis but OCD, depression, anxiety, substance misuse, and learning disability (Jayarajah 2025; Seeman 2014).

Many patients have told me they avoid disclosing their OCD to health professionals because they worry their fears will be misconstrued as facts. I see the difference between OCD and schizophrenia like chalk and cheese. On the surface, they may look similar but they are quite different. Below, I guide you through the hallmark features of psychoses and how they differ from OCD. Being able to decipher the difference between OCD and schizophrenia has huge implications for the patient's wellbeing, the consequential treatment options and management pathways, and potential need for safeguarding the patient's children and other family (Kimmel 2021).

Ego-syntonic or ego-dystonic thoughts?

To truly understand the concept of differential diagnosis between OCD and schizophrenia and related psychotic disorders (including postnatal psychosis), we need to take a closer look at the psychopathology (clinical study of mental disorders) and phenomenology (philosophical study of human experiences and consciousness). In simple terms, one can define ego-syntonic beliefs as beliefs that are in keeping with or the same (syntonic) as one's mind (ego), whereas ego-dystonic beliefs are beliefs that not in keeping with or different (dystonic) from one's mind (ego).

Through this lens, OCD can be characterised by thoughts and beliefs that are often grossly against the moral and ideological principles of the person. In this way, OCD would be considered an ego-dystonic thought process with ego-dystonic consequences. For example, a mother may have unwanted, intrusive, disturbing thoughts that the knife she's using to prepare dinner may slip from her hand and stab the baby next to her in the bouncer. She may be tormented by these thoughts, having visual and graphic images of her baby covered in blood because of her incompetence. She is quickly able to distance herself from the illness when asked about these thoughts, saying how 'frightened' and/or 'disgusted' she is by them. Some go so far as to say how alien and 'unlike me' the thoughts are.

In contrast, schizophrenia and related psychotic disorders are traditionally considered to consist of ego-syntonic beliefs. In the throes of mental illness, the dark, distressing thoughts become one with one's own thought process, which is characteristic of delusions. Consider the scenario above. In that situation, a mother experiencing psychosis post-delivery may have ego-syntonic thoughts that the devil possesses her baby, compelling her to harm the child with the knife in her hand. She may even be experiencing voices commanding her to act on these thoughts. Despite the ego-syntonic nature of the thoughts, many mothers who have experienced psychosis are able to hold onto their maternal caregiving instinct along with a deeper sense of wrong, resisting such dark thoughts, even when struggling with severe illness.

The level of insight and reflection on the situation really sets OCD and psychotic experiences apart. Maternal OCD might start her disclosure with phrases like *'I know this is stupid, but...'* or *'I know it sounds ridiculous, but I can't help having this fear that...'*. This level of insight rarely occurs in those experiencing acute psychosis or a schizophrenic relapse. In fact, these women often hold tightly to their beliefs, sometimes even trying to persuade others to believe them as well, citing specific signs or references that support their upsetting thoughts. For example, they might say, *'The midwife gave me a look and said, "What a lovely baby."'* and then add, *'That's when I knew she was trying to steal my newborn.'*

This is not to say that perinatal OCD is without risk. She may find her thoughts so overwhelming and distressing that they lead to low mood. In extreme cases, the intrusive thoughts and images can lead to thoughts of self-harm or a desire to end her life if she cannot see a way forward or out of the torment.

Sadly, women are often shamed for disclosure of any negative thoughts in the postnatal period, thus many are reluctant to share their intrusive thoughts with professionals. There is also a real fear about being sectioned under the Mental Health Act and/or having their children removed by social services. The likelihood of this happening for a woman with OCD is very low; however, the fear remains and will continue until there is a better understanding of OCD and ways to treat it.

Postnatal psychosis

Postnatal psychosis is a relatively rare condition, affecting approximately one in 1000 women. Those with a past history of psychotic-related disorders have a much higher risk of relapse, particularly if they have stopped medication during their pregnancy (which is common, as many women worry about medication effects on the developing foetus). Conditions such as bipolar disorder, schizophrenia, psychosis, and schizo-affective disorder all have the potential to escalate post-delivery and present as a postnatal psychosis. Even postnatal depression (although strictly not categorised as a psychotic illness) can have the potential to worsen and develop psychotic features in severe cases post-birth if left untreated.

Although we are still not clear on the exact causes of postnatal psychosis, we are aware that its likelihood of occurring is influenced by stressors, including perceived traumatic birth experience, sleep deprivation, low mood in relation to stress around newborn feeding issues, and family/external stressors.

Postnatal psychosis remains one of the few psychiatric emergencies in the speciality. It requires urgent and prompt attention and treatment, as women can deteriorate within a matter of hours (not weeks or months which is usually the case in first episode or relapses of psychosis presenting in the general population). The intrusive thoughts in postnatal psychosis are often paranoid in nature, thus the patient may be wary of health professionals, as well as friends and family members. There may also be a sudden change in their interactions and bond with the child – they may become overly protective to the point of smothering, or in contrast be suspicious of the child, believing that they are 'not theirs' or 'evil'.

Delusional beliefs are often coupled with experience of auditory hallucinations. The beliefs are so strong, they can tip women over the edge and cause them to act in drastic and unexpected ways, such as trying to jump out of the maternity ward window, trying to harm the baby in some way, or running away from the hospital after delivery with their infant (or indeed leaving the baby behind and absconding alone). As the risks in these cases are often high and unpredictable, special measures need to be put in place to ensure the safety of not only the mother but also the child. Special considerations in the management and treatment of postnatal psychosis are discussed in detail in Chapter 15.

OBJECTS OF DESIRE: STALKING, HARASSMENT, AND OCD

As previously discussed, OCD is characterised by unwanted, intrusive thoughts and/or images of an ego-dystonic nature. However, in stalking, the term 'obsession' relates to its alternative definition: frequent and overvalued thoughts of desire. This definition is more akin to the diagnosis of erotomania, defined as a delusional disorder where the individual (usually a woman) has a strongly held belief that the person (usually in a position of authority over her) is in love with her (Marazziti et al. 2015).

While stalking became high profile in 1990s mainstream culture through the obsession with celebrities, it is now recognised that social media plays a significant role in both the frequency and accessibility of stalking and harassment, which can occur in person or online (Faden et al. 2017). These kinds of obsessional thoughts are ego-syntonic, bringing the individual pleasure (as opposed to the significant personal suffering caused by these thoughts in OCD). Stalking perpetrators may even exhibit distorted beliefs and 'magical thinking' that not only suggest that someone, for example, their doctor, might be interested in them romantically, but also that through harassment and related behaviours they can influence the person' s mind, leading the person to fall madly in love with them. It is important to note that those working in mental health settings, particularly psychiatrists, psychologists, and psychotherapists, are especially vulnerable to becoming victims of stalking (Royal College of Psychiatrists 2023b). This is usually from a patient with a history of mental illness who is vulnerable to interpreting empathy as a sign of romantic connection or sexual attraction from the health professional. Health professionals are also at risk of being stalked at work by their ex-partners or people they know personally (Signori et al. 2022).

ADDICTIONS, IMPULSIVITY, AND PARAPHILIAS

Alcoholism, substance misuse, pathological gambling, and psychosexual disorders (paraphilias and non-paraphilic sex addiction) share the common theme of difficulty with control and impulsivity. People may engage in behaviours or experience violent and/or sexual urges but claim this is an 'illness' or due to a mental health condition such as OCD. This is a concern not only for the individual but also for how OCD and similar presentations are viewed and managed, especially in criminal and forensic contexts. In this next section we will explore each in detail and its relationship to OCD in the perinatal period.

Alcohol and drug addiction

People affected by alcohol and drug addiction often say they are obsessed with their substance or behaviour. In OCD, individuals are usually harm-avoidant, as obsessional thoughts and urges generate fear, and compulsive behaviours serve to reduce that fear. Conversely, in impulsivity disorders, people experience a drive and urge to seek out their compulsive behaviours, motivated by the anticipation of pleasure or the desire to lessen the anxious urge for their substance of choice – without the paralysing fear that something catastrophic would happen if they could not.

Coming back to our original definition of an obsession, in OCD, the thoughts are ego-dystonic, whereas in addictive and impulsive difficulties, the thoughts are usually ego-syntonic. Of course, one might not like or enjoy the feeling of being addicted. Once dependence takes hold, the addiction and related behaviours may no longer be pleasurable but necessary to function, thus becoming ego-dystonic in nature. Those affected may find themselves stuck in a vicious cycle, which can become harmful and potentially damaging to relationships, work, and quality of life, similar to what we see in severe OCD.

Another important overlap between OCD and addictions relates to using alcohol and other drugs (prescribed, over-the-counter, or illicit substances) to self-medicate and soothe the intense anxiety and distress caused by obsessions, aiming to alleviate symptoms. However, some drugs, such as cocaine, can worsen OCD symptoms. Due to the comorbidity of the two conditions, it is crucial to ask patients about alcohol and substance misuse, particularly during the perinatal period, as this can have damaging effects on foetal development, increasing the risk of congenital malformations, miscarriage, and stillbirth. Although mothers may initially feel motivated to abstain from substances during pregnancy, the likelihood of relapse after delivery remains high. The Royal College of Psychiatrists have recently published an extensive report for recommendations on co-occurring substance misuse and mental health disorders, recognising the complexities in supporting these patients and that services fail to recognise their additional needs (Royal College of Psychiatrists 2025).

Paraphilia disorder

Paraphilias (previously known as sexual perversions or sexual deviances) can be defined as recurrent, intense sexually arousing fantasies, sexual urges, or behaviours generally involving (a) non-human objects, (b) the suffering or humiliation of oneself or one's partner, or (c) children or other non-consenting persons that occur over a period of at least six months (McManus et al. 2013).

The DSM-5 now distinguishes between paraphilia and paraphiliac disorders, the key difference being the latter does not include the consent of an adult and/or inflicts pain or distress on the other individual. Examples include:

- exhibitionistic disorder (sexual arousal through exposing one's genitals or sexual organs to a non-consenting person)
- voyeuristic disorder (sexual arousal from watching others when they are naked or engaged in sexual activity)
- paedophilic disorder (primary or exclusive sexual attraction to prepubescent children).

Violent or aggressive sexual acts, such as molestation, sexual assault, and rape, can also trigger a sexually related OCD thought, but are not classified as sexual deviances, but rather sexual offences, and thus not a disorder but a criminal act (Kuty-Pachecka 2021).

As outlined in Chapter 3, understanding the SEXUAL/RELATIONSHIP OCD theme is particularly important in perinatal OCD as the parent in question may be the primary caregiver and responsible for the baby. Should there be symptoms of SEXUAL/RELATIONSHIP OCD, they may impact the child in a variety of ways, including:

- reduced bonding and attachment
- avoidance of the child (allowing other family members to take care of the baby, or neglect if limited support is available)
- avoidance of breastfeeding
- avoidance of attending to the daily care needs of the baby, such

as bathing or clothing them to avoid seeing and/or touching baby's genitals.

SEXUAL/RELATIONSHIP OCD can affect both fathers and mothers. It may strain the relationship and influence family dynamics during the perinatal period, which is recognised as a challenging time for couples caring for young children.

Health professionals and those working within the criminal justice system must understand the differences between SEXUAL/RELATIONSHIP OCD, sexual deviances, and sexual offences, as the management of each differs significantly. Getting it wrong can lead to long-lasting and serious consequences (Bradford 1999).

The distinction is crucial in managing perinatal OCD. Intrusive, unwanted sexual thoughts – such as believing that one might be a paedophile, could expose themselves inappropriately, or might become aroused whilst breastfeeding – are common but rarely disclosed fears in OCD clinics. For instance, a patient with such fears often tries everything to resist these thoughts, avoiding situations or places that could trigger them (e.g. playdates, children's birthday parties), or choosing to bottle feed instead of breastfeeding. The effort to suppress sexual obsessional thoughts usually fails, creating a vicious cycle of increasing obsessional ideas, known as 'the thought suppression paradox'.

Sexual compulsions can involve physically or mentally checking for arousal cues, intensely focusing on praying multiple times a day, and engaging in other religious practices, such as counting prayer beads. These acts are performed to counter what individuals perceive as inappropriate sexual thoughts and to demonstrate that they are moral and good people (Vella-Zarb et al. 2017).

Sexual thoughts in OCD are very distressing, and the person with SEXUAL/RELATIONSHIP OCD has no desire to act on these thoughts. Their aim is to stop thinking about them, as these thoughts cause significant distress and feelings of shame, guilt, and worry that they are a bad person. Sadly, I have frequently observed a lack of understanding about unwanted obsessional thoughts in clinical settings. Fear and confusion often lead health professionals to involve safeguarding or social services, or even calling the police, as the symptoms of OCD can be confused with sexual perversion.

TRAUMA IN THE PERINATAL PERIOD

Trauma during the perinatal period can significantly impact maternal mental health, often overlapping with conditions such as obsessive-compulsive disorder (OCD). As discussed in Chapter 1, intrusive thoughts, a key feature of perinatal OCD, may be worsened by the stress and unpredictability of labour. Patients with OCD (whether newly diagnosed or previously known) and/or a prior traumatic birth experience may also engage in more compulsive behaviours, such as requesting frequent investigations (e.g. repeated pelvic ultrasound scans) or specialist reviews for reassurance. Individuals concerned about birth trauma, much like those with perinatal OCD, might not find reassurance through repeated testing and could remain anxious throughout the perinatal period, which can be challenging for clinicians to manage (Mamun et al. 2023).

When birth experiences include factors such as loss of control, emergency interventions, or lack of support, it can lead to birth trauma and, in some cases, post-traumatic stress disorder (Brewin et al. 2025). The psychological effects may extend beyond the individual; unresolved trauma can influence parenting relationships, behaviours, and infant attachment (Ayers, Eagle, & Waring 2006). This can contribute to intergenerational trauma that may affect the child's emotional development. Addressing perinatal trauma comprehensively is therefore essential for both maternal wellbeing and the long-term health of the family unit. Although there are several potential avenues for trauma to develop in a woman's lifetime, in this section, I have focused on three specific examples of trauma that may be experienced in the perinatal period that have a close relationship to perinatal OCD:

- birth trauma
- post-traumatic stress disorder
- intergenerational trauma.

Birth trauma

Expectant parents prepare for a highly anticipated yet potentially challenging period with their newborn. While fear of the birth itself is quite common, the possibility of the birth becoming a traumatic event probably does not cross their minds, in keeping with what we have previously discussed in Part 2 of the idealisation of motherhood.

Those with diagnosed OCD and/or perfectionism traits may also struggle with this transition, as pregnancy and delivery represent events outside the parameters of predictability and control.

The UK Birth Trauma Association describes birth trauma as a commonly used term to describe the symptoms of distress a parent might experience after having gone through or witnessed a traumatic birth (Birth Trauma Association n.d.). It's important to remember that, as with other types of traumas not related to perinatal issues, the event simply needs to be perceived as traumatic by the person involved. Even if the birth went smoothly without any complications, a woman or her partner might still find themselves traumatised by what happened. Those with a history of adverse childhood events (such as sexual or physical abuse, emotional neglect, bullying, or household dysfunction) are more at risk of developing both physical and mental health problems during pregnancy (Tran et al. 2022). A large Australian study recently published also revealed that, beyond the well-known connection between maternal exposure to adverse childhood experiences and perinatal anxiety and depression, these women are almost four times more likely to perceive their birth experience as traumatic (Mackle et al. 2023). In some cases the birth complications and stress related to this event may result in post-traumatic stress disorder.

Post-traumatic stress disorder

Although post-traumatic stress disorder (PTSD) was officially recognised as a diagnosis in 1980, its signs and symptoms have been acknowledged for over 3000 years. Ancient descriptions of war-related trauma, inscribed in stone, noted psychological and physical symptoms that still define trauma today. In the past, trauma was linked to female 'hysteria' (as mentioned in Chapter 7) – women were believed to be 'weak' because of their womb. Neuroscientists later associated negative experiences with changes in the brain, especially emphasising how war and conflict impact the nervous system. We now know that there is a delicate balance of chemical and hormonal changes (specifically the ovarian steroid hormones oestrogen and progesterone along with the neurosteroid allopregnanolone) that make women more susceptible to the effects of psychological stress and traumatic events. In fact, women are twice as likely as men to experience PTSD and have a greater prevalence of comorbid mental health disorders compared with men (Ravi, Stevens, & Michopoulos 2019).

It is estimated that approximately 4% of women will experience PTSD after childbirth. Psychologists at the University of Sussex have found that a history of depression, tokophobia, or previous PTSD increases the risk of developing postnatal PTSD. Risk factors during or after birth for PTSD include having a negative subjective experience of labour, undergoing an assisted vaginal delivery or caesarean section, and lacking support (Ayers et al. 2016).

OCD shares similarities with PTSD in that both conditions can present in a very physical/medicalised way. In both conditions, individuals may experience preoccupation with an event, along with repeated unwanted intrusive thoughts and images. In PTSD, the literature often refers to these experiences as 'flashbacks', noting a distressing and unwanted memory from the past (such as the experience of being in a car crash) intruding into the present as if the event were happening in the present rather than in the past. By contrast, in OCD, patients experience a 'flash-forward'. They may have a distressing and unwanted intrusive thought or image, but it is often a worst-case scenario about something that could happen in the future, rather than bringing back something that has happened to them in the past. Using the car crash analogy, those with perinatal OCD might describe having intense worries with intrusive images of being in a car crash, specifically seeing their child covered in blood and glass on the side of the road (Grekin, O'Hara, & Brock 2021).

'What happens if it actually happens?' Confirmation of fears

With perinatal OCD, the challenge in clinical practice occurs when the fear becomes real. I once had a patient who experienced intrusive, unwanted thoughts and images about harm coming to her baby boy; for example, that she might accidentally drop him. She continued the prescribed treatment, which included a combination of psychological therapy and medication. She showed some initial improvements until she accidentally dropped her baby. Thankfully, he was fine, and there were no concerns about his health from the incident. The mother experienced a complex set of emotions – initially she was very distressed that her fears had materialised, but she was relieved that her worst fears of him dying did not happen. Through therapeutic work, she was able to incorporate this traumatic experience into her recovery.

When this occurs, it is often a pivotal and defining moment in the treatment progression. However, it is difficult to predict how someone will react. For some, it offers a reality check and a sense of relief; they can see objectively that, despite their worst fears coming true, they were able to survive, showing that what actually happened was not as catastrophic as they had imagined. Such an event can foster a newfound confidence in their recovery goals. Conversely, others might find the realisation of their worst fears becoming reality overwhelming, which can worsen their OCD symptoms and hinder their progress in treatment.

Intergenerational trauma

Intergenerational trauma refers to the passing of trauma effects from one generation to the next. Many communities worldwide have experienced collective traumas, which create the potential for intergenerational trauma. War, civil unrest, natural disasters, economic and political crises, migration, seeking asylum, and sexual or racial discrimination are just some examples of how personal and social circumstances can shape experiences and become embedded in stories passed down through generations. The transmission can occur through various mechanisms, such as changes in gene expression or influencing parenting behaviours. The perinatal period is a sensitive time for inheriting or expressing intergenerational trauma, as it can have long-lasting effects on the parent–infant relationship (Yehuda & Lehrner 2018).

Understanding intergenerational trauma is vital for those working in towns and cities that are melting pots of cultures with immigrant communities from various backgrounds. This also applies to people born and raised in the UK but whose parents and grandparents come from different countries, meaning they might (consciously or subconsciously) pass on ideas and traumas from their own migration experiences. These can be intentional, like retelling past traumatic events, or subconscious, such as their fearful, overprotective behaviour or mistrust of others that originate from previous experiences.

Intergenerational trauma can also extend beyond the birth experience, involving psychosocial and cultural aspects of historical trauma. Complex thoughts and feelings about identity and culture often surface with the birth of a baby, as the event may trigger a range of (mostly unconscious or repressed) emotions linked to their culture. This is also true for couples raising children of dual heritage or mixed race, who must decide on certain traditions (religious, cultural, and familial) when bringing up their child. As discussed previously, it is vital to be familiar with the cultural and social context of one's experiences of OCD and their perceptions of traumatic experience.

OCD AND PERSONALITY DISORDERS

Although perfectionism is common among both mothers and individuals with OCD during the perinatal period, recognising the difference between having a perfectionist personality trait and a personality disorder is important. The two manuals ICD-11 and DSM-5 classify different types or clusters of personality disorders. Types include emotionally unstable, narcissistic, and antisocial. Technically, any parent could exhibit any variations in personality structure and subsequent disorder on the severe end of the personality disorder spectrum. However, a noted special relationship exists between perinatal OCD and obsessive-compulsive personality disorder (OCPD), also known as anankastic personality disorder.[2]

In anankastic personality disorder, the main concerns are perfectionism, order, and cleanliness. Rigid thinking is also a characteristic and differs from that seen in OCD. People with this disorder appear inflexible and need total control over tasks, micromanaging through endless lists and projects. They also exhibit obsessive attention to detail and insist on adhering to rules and regulations, despite others' suggestions. They often resist change and are inflexible in their interactions with others. Unlike individuals with OCD, they are not

2 I use 'anankastic personality disorder' for ease of reference and to avoid the confusion many experience between OCD and OCPD.

troubled by others' opinions of them and remain committed to their own beliefs, ideas, and expectations. They seek little to no reassurance from others.

As discussed earlier in the book, severe perfectionism and anankastic personality disorder are very difficult to manage. In the workplace, perfectionism can become paralysing, as someone with the disorder will not be able to finish a project until it is perfect. In the perinatal period, it can influence their views on the pregnancy and birth experience, as well as their relationship with healthcare providers. Treatment may be a difficult topic to broach, as those who have anankastic personality disorder typically do not think they have a 'problem' to begin with, and are more likely to blame the situation on others' incompetence. They respond well to a cognitive behavioural therapy approach, should they choose to take part in treatment, which we will discuss more in Chapter 16.

In conclusion, the overview of differential diagnoses allows for more accurate assessment and identification of perinatal OCD. Particularly when working in specialist perinatal mental health services, one must be mindful of dual diagnosis and how the presentation may be complicated, impacting both the mother and child/unborn. In Part 5, I summarise the treatment pathways of perinatal OCD.

PART 5

TREATING PERINATAL OCD

In this final part of the book, I look at the various treatment options for perinatal OCD, with reference to the unique aspects of the condition that benefit from specialist support during pregnancy and the postpartum period. As mentioned previously, there is separate guidance on OCD treatment, and guidance on treating perinatal mental health disorders, but no specific consensus on national guidance for the niche subspeciality of perinatal OCD in the UK. The information available is often grouped under the umbrella of anxiety disorders in the postnatal period, or pre-existing OCD or anxiety disorders in women who become pregnant. The following chapters are not a substitute for referral but rather provide an overview of services and treatments currently available in the UK.

In Chapter 14, I summarise the relevant national guidance for OCD and management of antenatal and postnatal mental health and explain the makeup of the perinatal mental health service and standard referral process. In Chapter 15, I categorise treatment options based on location (inpatient or outpatient), usually dependent on severity, need, and patient preferences, highlighting the 'red flag' symptoms to be aware of in severe perinatal mental illness. Although hospital admission is quite rare for the treatment of perinatal OCD, I summarise the options available, including the specialist mother and baby units that might be a viable option to avoid parent–infant separation at a vulnerable time. Though I do not explicitly discuss this in the book, another dimension to consider is choosing where to access treatment for their perinatal OCD, specifically deciding whether to go through the NHS or the private sector. This book predominantly focuses on treatment within the UK national healthcare system. However, it is important to note that with the increased demand for consultations via the private sector, the same principles apply, and the guidance will serve those practising across NHS and private care. Chapter 16 summarises the psychological therapies, family approaches, creative arts, and the medications that may be helpful in the treatment of perinatal OCD[1] with special reference to unique considerations to be mindful of in the perinatal period, such as medication use in pregnancy and breastfeeding. I conclude Part 5 with an overview of new treatments on the horizon. Neuromodulation techniques, such as deep brain stimulation (DBS) and transcranial magnetic stimulation (TMS), continue to cause quite a stir in neuroscientific circles and appear to be a promising future therapeutic option.

1 Unless specified the treatments outlined in this book focus on the adult treatment of perinatal OCD, not the treatment of children or young adults, who would be referred to and managed within child and adolescent mental health services (CAMHS).

CHAPTER 14

NICE Guidelines for OCD and Perinatal Mental Health

In this chapter, I share an overview of the current guidelines from the National Institute for Health and Care Excellence (NICE) for the best practices in OCD treatment. I also look at how best to manage both OCD and perinatal mental health conditions within NHS settings.

NICE GUIDELINES

NICE guidelines provide national guidance and advice to health professionals to improve health and social care, through evidence-based recommendations led by an expert panel with patient involvement. NICE was created in 1999, with the first clinical guidelines published in 2002 on the management of schizophrenia. They cover a wide range of topics pertinent to clinical practice, including guidance on assessing physical and mental health conditions, the use of diagnostic tests, public health advice, and treatment recommendations. Currently, there are no written guidelines specifically for the assessment, management, and treatment of perinatal OCD. In this chapter, I will summarise the key findings from the two relevant reports:[1]

1 The guideline 'Obsessive-compulsive disorder and body dysmorphic disorder: Assessment and management' is currently in development with publication date to be confirmed.

- CG31: Obsessive-compulsive disorder and body dysmorphic disorder: Treatment (NICE 2005)
- CG192: Antenatal and postnatal mental health: Clinical management and service guidance (NICE 2014, last updated February 2020).

NICE recommendations for OCD treatment and assessment of perinatal mental health

Patients may delay seeking help and support not only because of the stigma surrounding mental health but also due to the shame and embarrassment linked to revealing their OCD symptoms. The guidelines recognise that many people refrain from seeking help because the less common intrusive thoughts about sexual aggression or death are often misunderstood as signs of risk. This is especially true in perinatal environments, where mothers might experience unwanted intrusive thoughts about their baby, worry about being misunderstood by professionals, and fear that disclosing such thoughts could lead to a referral to children's social services, risking the removal of their child.

The guidance advises that all NHS trusts should have dedicated specialist mental health services staffed with skilled health professionals who are proficient in recognising and treating OCD. They advise on developing services using a stepped-care model approach. This approach provides a framework of working that is inclusive of the different needs of people with OCD, allowing timely access and effective interventions to be offered. As steps 1 and 2 have previously been discussed in Chapter 12, I will be focusing on steps 3–6 in this final part of the book.

- Step 1: awareness and recognition
- Step 2: recognition and assessment
- Steps 3–5: treatment options for people with OCD or BDD
- Step 6: intensive treatment and inpatient services for people with OCD or BDD.

CG192 offers a specialised overview of the principles of care during pregnancy and the postnatal period. It emphasises the importance of supporting women, their partners, families, and carers – especially young women and those with known mental health disorders. The document recommends that services provide coordinated care, which is especially vital in the perinatal period as families may access multiple services (such as midwifery, health visiting, mental health services, and social care). The guidelines summarise the evidence base for the management and treatment of common mental health conditions, such as postnatal depression and anxiety, but unfortunately do not explicitly mention perinatal OCD. Similarly, the OCD guidelines do not specifically address perinatal OCD; however, we hope that, through advocacy from the charity Maternal OCD and other organisations, this will be included in future updates. In clinical practice, we integrate the recommendations from both reports to customise the assessment, treatment, and management offered through our specialist services.

A holistic approach to treatment options in perinatal OCD must consider the biological, psychological, and social aspects of recovery. For example, a mother of four children who is recovering from a traumatic birth experience may be hesitant to be admitted to a mother and baby unit, as she will be separated from her older children and family support. Another common scenario we observe in clinical practice is a patient with OCD who is eager to engage in therapy but finds it difficult to leave the house and attend the clinic due to overwhelming obsessions and compulsive behaviours.

We can further subcategorise current treatment options by:

- duration (short-term/long-term management)
- location (community/ward)
- mode of treatment (broadly divided into psychological and pharmacological)
- severity of illness and/or comorbid conditions.

The most common pathway in the UK for management of perinatal OCD is via referral to the local psychological and/or perinatal mental health services, which I outline below.

PERINATAL MENTAL HEALTH SERVICES

As part of NHS England's long-term plan, the Five Year Forward View for Mental Health made a commitment to transform perinatal mental health services across England (NHS England 2016; NHS Mental

Health Taskforce 2016). With an injection of over two billion pounds, it promised that by 2023/24, at least 66,000 women with moderate, complex, or severe perinatal mental health needs could access timely care and support in the community.[2] This, coupled with additional funding and transformation of maternity services, aims to boost recognition and timely intervention for women with mental health conditions in pregnancy as well as support when planning a pregnancy (NHS England n.d.). It is important to understand exactly what you can expect when making a referral, especially if you are working in services outside of mental health and are unsure of what the service entails.

Perinatal mental health services are multidisciplinary teams that focus on caring for the mental health needs of women and their children during pregnancy and the postnatal period. At the time of writing this, however, both the inclusion criteria and the definition of the postnatal period are undergoing changes in services across the country. Traditionally, community and inpatient perinatal mental health services support women for up to one year postnatal, but many services have already extended this to two years. Some services have also begun integrating services by developing '0–5-year-olds' hubs. This is part of the government's vision to improve the mental health of children and young people, coupled with the recognition of the importance of early childhood and infant mental health (Royal College of Psychiatrists 2023a).

Perinatal mental health team members

The perinatal mental health team is made up of different health professionals, all of whom have a specialist interest and knowledge in working with women and babies during the perinatal period. Most teams will have perinatal psychiatrists, perinatal psychologists, perinatal psychiatric nurses, occupational therapists, social workers, and administrative staff. Additional staff members may include nursery nurses and parent–infant psychotherapists.

External to the team, but working closely, are midwives, health visitors, and neonatal staff who may have an additional interest in

2 The target of 66,000 women accessing timely care was previously set in the NHS Mental Health Implementation plan 2019/20 – 2023/24, which was a continuation of the Five Year Forward view for mental health report (2016).

perinatal mental health. Most perinatal services are more than happy to welcome trainees from all disciplines who want to gain additional insight and expertise in working in the subspeciality. Unlike the traditional medical model, in mental health settings, almost all the healthcare professionals listed above can and will conduct initial assessments and review patients in the hospital or community, not just the psychiatrist or resident doctor.

Who can be referred

It is predominantly mothers (both biological and non-biological) and those attempting to conceive who are referred to us. However, there is a shift towards including fathers and/or partners, as increasing evidence shows that partners also experience mental illness during the perinatal period. As discussed previously, any caregiver with OCD can affect the children and family. Being more inclusive in supporting partners and/or fathers through services and treatment is vital for improving overall family wellbeing.

One must, however, be mindful of factors such as team resources, case-load burden, patient confidentiality, and safeguarding concerns – for example, if there is a past or current history of intimate partner violence. The charity Women's Aid reports that 20–30% of postnatal women will experience violence from a partner/ex-partner during pregnancy and that domestic violence may begin or escalate during or after the pregnancy (Women's Aid 2019).

On making a referral to a perinatal mental health service, the main consideration is the need to provide support to women with mental illness difficulties, either pre-dating the pregnancy or new onset in the pregnancy/postnatal period. Other considerations include concerns about bonding and attachment with the baby (including reduced bonding, if noted during pregnancy), worries about the birth process, and mood difficulties surrounding traumatic or complicated deliveries.

Special considerations for dual diagnosis – OCD and neurodiversity

Perinatal OCD can often occur alongside other conditions, such as depression (National Autistic Society, n.d.). As discussed in previous chapters, it is important to recognise that the standardised assessment and treatment options may require additional attention in dual diagnosis. Those with a dual diagnosis of OCD and autism spectrum disorder (ASD) may benefit from psychological interventions to tackle intrusive and repetitive thoughts and behaviours.[3] It is important to note a key difference, however, that with regard to medication use in the perinatal period, those with perinatal OCD often report real improvement when titrating dose to maximum dosage. In contrast, those with an autism diagnosis are very sensitive to side effects and tolerate only minimal dosing of psychotropic medication.

Those on the neurodivergent spectrum may benefit from personalised care throughout pregnancy and postpartum, with tailored support identifying their specific needs and challenges early on. They may benefit from additional social support through charities that help mothers and babies, as well as streamlined care from maternity with a named midwife/health visitor who provides continuity of care to reduce feelings of anxiety and overwhelm from seeing different member of staff at each appointment.

---

3 Autism spectrum disorder is the diagnostic term for autism. However, it's important to be aware that many people prefer to use identify first language (autistic person) rather than 'with autism' or 'ASD'. Clinicians should take care to consult those they interact with on their preference.

CHAPTER 15

Outpatient and Inpatient Treatment

Depending on patient preference, severity of symptoms, and clinical need, the treatment of OCD in the perinatal period can occur at home, in a community clinic, or after admission to hospital. I summarise the options available, before highlighting the warning signs that would warrant consideration for an inpatient admission or crisis support.

COMMUNITY (OUTPATIENT) TREATMENT

For the most part, perinatal OCD is a condition that can be managed almost exclusively in a community setting through a combination of consistent, longer-term psychological and pharmacological intervention (see Chapter 16). Many of our patients do not make it through the doors of secondary-care specialist services, as their perinatal OCD is adequately addressed by those working in primary care, namely GPs and psychologists as part of talking therapies.

Depending on where you live, psychological services may have different names, such as 'talking therapies' or 'IAPT' (improving access to psychological therapies). Essentially, each offers community-based psychological services aligned with primary-care settings. They provide a range of psychological interventions for mild to moderate mental health issues, such as phobias, anxiety disorder, and OCD. The services offered are often time-limited (six to twelve sessions), and those providing treatment may not have specific expertise in working with women and/or perinatal OCD.

Most talking-therapy services will provide a generic cognitive behavioural therapy approach. Many will offer a range of psychological therapies. such as group therapy or psychodynamic psychotherapy. For treatment of OCD, cognitive behavioural therapy (CBT) for OCD, or exposure and response prevention therapy (an advanced type of cognitive behavioural therapy used specifically for OCD treatment), is offered as first line and is recommended by NICE guidance for community treatment (NICE 2005).

Many primary care psychological services have expanded to provide specific support for women in pregnancy and the postnatal period. They may offer support groups and trained professionals to manage conditions such as postnatal anxiety and depression or birth trauma. This aligns with the perspective that women, parents, and families benefit from access to specialised services that support their unique needs (Stevens et al. 2018).

NICE guidelines for antenatal and postnatal mental health and for OCD recognise the importance of treatment provided by clinicians with more expertise in specialist settings (NICE 2005, 2014). For mild and/or first presentations of mild OCD where the impact on quality of life and daily functioning is minimal, low-intensity (up to ten hours) psychological therapy can be beneficial. This can take the form of self-guided CBT, telephone (virtual) CBT, or group CBT. For moderate OCD presentation and/or those who have not responded to limited psychological therapy, one can consider more intensive CBT (more than ten hours of therapy) or the addition of medication (preferably an SSRI antidepressant). In severe OCD, NICE guidelines recommend combination treatment of medication and psychological intervention (including exposure and response prevention therapy). As previously discussed, individuals with perinatal OCD may encounter unique challenges not typically experienced by the general, non-perinatal population, which can make accessing therapy more difficult. For example, they may be housebound or need to arrange childcare in order to attend appointments. To address these challenges, many perinatal mental health services have embraced an integrated community care approach, outlined below.

Integrated community care

Integrated community clinics aligned with other services (such as maternity, health visiting, or school) are excellent family-friendly places to access care. One of the benefits of hosting clinics in children's centres is that it immediately makes services more accessible and removes the stigma associated with going to a psychiatric unit or mental health clinic. It also provides a safe space for children to play, learn, and grow, and a place for mothers to rest and feel supported in their parenting. These centres offer one-to-one peer support, a variety of groups (such as stay and play, music time, or baby massage), as well as support from infant-feeding coordinators and children centre practitioners. Practitioners may provide support in getting to and from the centre or a listening ear giving advice about concerns around sleep routine, teething, or other common dilemmas of the first years of becoming a parent.

It is also a lot more practical for service users to get to, as these community children centres are dotted around the borough and by their very nature are baby-friendly. This feature makes a huge difference to parents in the perinatal period. Women can often walk to these centres or have a short journey to them, without worrying about hospital parking or the logistics of taking a baby to hospital. This increases engagement with services and reduces 'did not attend' and appointment cancellations.

The royal stamp of approval

In November 2022, our perinatal mental health service received a visit from Her Royal Highness, the Princess of Wales. In her new role as Patron of the Maternal Mental Health Alliance, she was keen to visit a community perinatal team. Our service is unique for its integrated model of community care, created over time through mutual respect and trust between the NHS, local authority, and charity sectors.

That day, I led a round-table discussion around improving perinatal mental healthcare for women and wellbeing for families. Staff from maternity, perinatal mental health teams, talking therapies, health visiting, and charity organisations contributed to the discussions. We talked about the strengths of inter-agency working but also the challenges we face in the community, particularly the stigma mothers continue to face around accessing perinatal mental health support. The visit was held at a local children centre (separate from our NHS clinics), where we run some of our postnatal clinics, which are a lifeline for mothers and parents during pregnancy and the early years. The Princess of Wales was very knowledgeable about maternal mental health and quoted studies from Harvard University on child development. Her passion was infectious. Later, we were told she felt inspired by our work as a collective in the community. She has since launched the Early Childhood Foundation and has openly expressed that maternal mental health and the wellbeing of families is a future priority for her and the Royal Family.

HOSPITAL (INPATIENT) TREATMENT

As with all illnesses, both physical and mental, there may be occasions where community treatment is no longer a viable option. Perhaps the symptoms have become too debilitating, or the former community options have been exhausted, and the patient remains unwell to a degree that she may be unsafe to both herself and her baby, or for another equally valid reason. In these circumstances, one may consider hospital admission, either voluntarily or under the Mental Health Act, depending on the circumstances and nature/degree of the presentation.

Someone who over a long period of time has not responded to community interventions and/or has other conditions can be classified as having severe OCD. The risks to someone with severe OCD may be extreme distress, functional impairment, self-neglect and life threat. In these circumstances, it may be recommended that the individual comes into hospital for a period of assessment and treatment, ideally to a specialist unit for treatment of OCD and related disorders. However, before admission to a psychiatric unit, the patient must be medically fit and receive treatment for any illnesses that may be a sequela of their mental health. For example, if they are dehydrated, they must be given intravenous fluids and any other necessary treatment (dehydration is a common finding in those with severe OCD as they may restrict their fluid intake and eating).

The main benefits of hospital admission are:

- management of the acute risks with severe loss of function
- closer monitoring
- protection through having staff who can support, monitor, and help to reduce the risks identified to both mother and child.

At present in the UK under the NHS, four potential avenues for inpatient treatment exist for perinatal OCD, each of which has advantages and disadvantages:

- mother and baby psychiatric unit (MBU) where both mother and baby can be admitted together to access treatment and support
- general adult psychiatric ward (individual admission separated from infant)
- specialised adult OCD unit (will receive specialist treatment and intervention but will be separated from baby)
- perinatal OCD service as part of community mental health team which can be attended with baby.

Hospital admission

In an MBU admission the infant is admitted with the mother, an added benefit as it reduces the likelihood of maternal separation. In a general adult (also known as acute) mental health ward admission, the mother comes alone. This may be by choice or because the presentation is an acute crisis in keeping with severe and enduring mental illnesses.

With MBU or mental health ward admission, some find the environment of being with patients who have severe and enduring mental illness (such as postnatal psychosis or bipolar disorder) very distressing, as their symptoms and behaviours are very different compared to their perinatal OCD illness. As discussed previously, most women with maternal OCD who are admitted to a psychiatric inpatient unit come as a voluntary admission. This means they have the mental capacity and insight to make the decision and agree to come into hospital for treatment.

Some patients may be admitted under the Mental Health Act, but this is unlikely in the case of perinatal OCD. The patient's agency in making decisions about their care along with their motivation to engage in treatment is essential to the treatment and recovery processes of perinatal OCD. This is particularly important for psychological interventions, which are the mainstay of treatment in most cases. On rare occasions, I have seen women sectioned under the Mental Health Act for perinatal OCD because urgent intervention was needed for their safety and/or the safety of others. In these cases, their functioning was severely impaired by the rigidity of their beliefs and/or their perinatal OCD was comorbid with another illness, such as severe postnatal depression.

RISK ASSESSMENT

Deciding whether to start treatment in hospital or in the community can be a complex decision, but it always involves carefully considering the risks involved.

In perinatal services, we must be mindful of not only the risk to the mother but also risk to the baby, children, and others. During the risk assessment, the clinician must ascertain whether the unborn child and/or baby is at risk of harm or neglect. This may be in relation to the parent feeling paralysed by obsessional ruminations and/or being so preoccupied with performing OCD rituals that they are unable to attend to the baby's needs. Parents may also show evidence of neglect by not accessing care and treatments for their children because of their OCD beliefs. Should these concerns arise, it would warrant further review and consideration of children and safeguarding involvement, crisis support, and/or hospital admission. Although the signs described below can occur for anyone with perinatal mental illness, clinical risk scenarios to pay particular attention to in the pregnant or postnatal parent with OCD include:

- refusing to attend hospital appointments
- not permitting childhood immunisations
- going against recommendations by professionals to supplement with formula feeding/other treatments due to concerns about infant weight loss and failure to thrive
- older siblings not attending school or being late to school
- elaborate bathing routine for baby/children
- physical signs of irritated or dry skin in newborns, indicative of frequent washing or use of soaps/skin disinfectants

- frequent A&E/urgent-care presentations for medical concerns
- signs of emotional, psychological, or physical abuse, or neglect of children.

Postnatal psychosis: A psychiatric emergency

Postnatal psychosis is a psychiatric emergency that can be mistaken for postnatal OCD or can occur as a result of deteriorating mood and mental state in those experiencing depression, anxiety, or OCD. 'Red flag' signs include experiencing psychotic symptoms (such as paranoid thoughts, auditory or visual hallucinations), changes in mood, or new thoughts of self-harm, as well as estrangement from the baby.

If symptoms appear soon after delivery and the mother and baby remain on the maternity unit, an urgent mental health review should be requested on the ward, with consideration of one-to-one supervision by a trained health professional who will stay with the patient at all times, monitor their mental state, and administer medication (oral or injectable, if required). If there are serious concerns about the mother's treatment of the child, it may be advisable to temporarily separate the baby or nurse the mother on an open ward where interactions can be observed. However, some argue that this environment is already busy and stressful enough, so a side room might be preferred to minimise risks.

A safeguarding referral must be made to the children and family safeguarding team and social care to ensure the family receives support during this challenging time. If symptoms of psychosis occur in the community, with the patient at home with her baby and family, an urgent referral to crisis services should be made (not a general referral to a mental health team, which might take days or weeks to respond and offer an appointment). Crisis mental health services operate 24/7 and can provide specialist support and review outside usual hours.

Consideration should be given to admission to a psychiatric mother and baby unit (MBU), where mother and baby can be assessed and treated safely with supervision. Although hospital admission (especially to a mental health ward) may seem like a last resort, in perinatal mental health, early admission is often preferred, allowing the condition to be addressed before it affects the mother–baby bond, aiding recovery (Stephenson et al. 2018).

PSYCHIATRIC MOTHER AND BABY UNITS

To manage severe perinatal OCD (as well as other severe mental health conditions presenting in the perinatal period), NICE guidelines recommend psychiatric admission, ideally to a specialist MBU (NICE 2014). There are 22 such units across the UK. Three are based in London with six to ten beds per unit, highlighting the niche and specialist nature of these services. At present, these are NHS England funded services. Referrals are not dependent on patient address, meaning that beds are available across the UK irrespective of where a patient lives.

Patients can be admitted to an MBU by choice or voluntarily (often described as 'informally'), or formally through detention under the Mental Health Act. A recent study highlighted that mothers with mental health needs prefer overall to be admitted to MBUs with their baby. They are seen to be family-focused and offer more perinatal specialist expertise and treatment compared with a general mental health ward. It was also recognised that during this vulnerable period, maternal separation from their baby for treatment of their mental health crisis on an acute general ward could be a traumatic experience that may impact on recovery (Griffiths et al. 2019).

Once admitted to an MBU, patients can expect a longer admission (two to three months on average) than with acute mental health wards. On an MBU, they can access several treatment options and interventions, including individual psychological therapy, art therapy, music therapy, family therapy, and parent–infant psychotherapy. They also have regular medical and nursing reviews, with pharmacological treatment options considered alongside psychosocial interventions.

All MBUs have a nursery and nursery-nurse staff in addition to adult mental health nursing staff. This allows mothers to access childcare support whilst having treatment. Patients have the option of leaving the ward for a period, whether for a walk around the hospital grounds and/or going home to stay with family prior to being discharged from the unit.

The barriers affecting a patient's choice of hospital admission for perinatal OCD treatment are complex. Some reasons for declining admission relate to practical considerations, particularly if the mother has other children at home. MBUs accept admissions for babies up to one year postnatal and do not allow partners or siblings to be admitted. Additional challenges include being admitted far from home due to lack of local bed availability. Other concerns involve the mental health stigma and the emotional impact of being admitted during the postnatal period, which may trigger feelings of guilt or shame for seeking help. Other circumstances pertain to the admission eligibility criteria, for example presenting to services after the child's first birthday.

MBRRACE-UK (Mothers and Babies: Reducing Risk through Audits and Confidential Enquiries across the UK)

MBRRACE-UK, who are funded by the Healthcare Quality Improvement Partnership, undertake confidential enquiries into maternal morbidity and mortality, with reports being released annually. These reports detail all the causes of death in women who have died within a year of childbirth in the UK. Although the report recognises a few medical conditions contributing to the death of women in the postnatal period (e.g. cardiac disease, sepsis, stroke, and thrombosis), maternal suicide remains the leading direct cause of death occurring in the year following childbirth, and this saddening statistic has remained consistent since the MBRRACE-UK reports were first published in the 1980s.

Women who die by suicide during the perinatal period choose severe and violent methods, such as hanging, jumping off a bridge/in front of a train, or jumping from a building. In the most recent report published, nearly three-quarters of women who died had a pre-existing diagnosis of a physical or mental health condition, and 8% of women were identified as having multiple disadvantages, including a mental health diagnosis, substance misuse, and history of domestic violence.

CHAPTER 16

Therapies and Medications

In this chapter, we will take a deep dive into the nitty-gritty of what psychological therapy entails, including the theory and driving principles of how it works as a successful treatment modality, as well as an overview of the specialist adaptations for psychological therapy treatment specific to the perinatal period for OCD. I also touch on adjunctive therapies, such as family therapy and arts therapy, that may be helpful in managing the condition.

Finally, I hope to provide clarity on a complex aspect of care: the use of medication for treatment of perinatal OCD. This is a topic that brings up several questions and anxieties in clinical practice for patients and professionals alike, with the default status to discontinue medication for fear of causing accidental harm. I discuss special considerations when making decisions about taking medication during this vulnerable time and have created a summary table of common medications prescribed for the treatment of OCD, outlining the safety profile of each in pregnancy and breastfeeding. As mentioned before, the advice provided is a mere guide and will need a case-by-case approach. Where possible, I would recommend referral to a specialist psychiatrist who has experience in prescribing for OCD, and with additional expertise in prescribing under special considerations such as for those who are pregnant or breastfeeding.

PSYCHOLOGICAL TREATMENT OF OCD

Psychological (talking) therapies remain the mainstay of OCD treatment, as identified in the evidence-based literature, NICE guidelines, and in clinical practice (Reid et al. 2021). The good news is that perinatal OCD responds very well to timely and specific psychological interventions, allowing many patients to make a complete recovery. Exposure and response prevention (ERP), a specific type of cognitive behavioural therapy (discussed below), has had the best results for reducing symptom burden in OCD and is now considered the first choice for treatment.

The origins of cognitive behavioural therapy for OCD

In the early 20th century, OCD was predominantly treated through psychoanalytical and neurosurgical techniques. In psychoanalytical practice, as popularised by Sigmund Freud and discussed earlier in the book, the emphasis is on understanding how the unconscious mind influences conscious thoughts and behaviours. From the 1940s onwards, there was a move towards psychological therapies, specifically addressing not only cognitive theories but also the behavioural components of OCD. For OCD, much of the treatment rationale underpinning CBT originated from Mowrer's classic work on fear and avoidance, which involves two distinct stages – classical and operant conditioning (Mowrer & Lamoreaux 1946). He suggested that fear of thoughts, images, or objects is first acquired through a classical conditioning process in the first stage. In OCD, he contended, the trigger for symptoms is almost always related to a perceived traumatic event. In the second stage, the fear is maintained through operant conditioning, where behaviours can be modified depending on the outcome. Specifically, if something is perceived as a reward or a positive influence, it will promote the behaviour; if seen as a punishment or negative influence, it will reduce the behaviour.

A good example of Mower's theory is seen in day-to-day parenting. A child receives a reward for completing a certain behaviour (e.g. permission to play video games for completing their homework) or a punishment for negative behaviour, with the hope of reducing repetition of that behaviour (e.g. a child being placed in 'time out' after having a tantrum).

If we apply Mower's theory to perinatal OCD, common reactions to a fear could include avoidance, escapism, compulsions, or safety behaviours. They all aim to reinforce the desired outcome (fear reduction) in a positive way, so they will continue to be repeated. Safety behaviours may be subtle but are frequently seen in parents who do a variety of checks or other safety behaviours, often unconsciously, to ensure that their child is not in danger. Examples include checking the temperature of the bath water several times or avoiding bath times completely – delegating the task to their partner instead. In perinatal OCD, these safety mechanisms may be instinctual and signify both a sense of care and responsibility. However, one must be mindful whether this is indeed part of a bigger picture of an OCD presentation.

In OCD treatment, we aim to break the cycle of the positive reward mechanism associated with obsessional thinking and compulsive rituals. The goal is to reduce and stop compulsive behaviours by neutralising the fear that has restricted them. In a series of behavioural experiments during treatment, the therapist challenges the person with OCD to imagine or consider doing the opposite of their usual reaction to unwanted thoughts and images, thereby facing their fear and challenging their own assumptions head-on (with the support of a therapist).

Cognitive behavioural therapy

NICE guidelines place cognitive behavioural therapy (CBT) as the gold standard and a first-line evidence-based therapy for the treatment of OCD. CBT is an intervention that focuses on an individual's thoughts, feelings, and actions. It is believed that the three are interlinked: our thoughts (cognition) can affect our feelings which in turn govern our actions (behaviour). People can fall into negative thought cycles. In CBT the aim is to shift the core beliefs that shape our way of thinking, with the hope of exerting a better, more positive, influence on our feelings and subsequent actions.

CBT is used for a variety of mental health conditions, most commonly the treatment of anxiety or phobias, and can also be used to treat perinatal OCD. In traditional CBT, we begin to challenge negative beliefs and assumptions, whilst also taking small steps towards overcoming the fears and slowly shifting the end behaviour. It requires a step-by-step approach so the patient doesn't become overwhelmed by doing too much too quickly. Regular check-ins with the patient and reassurance (within reason) is required to ensure that the therapy is done in a safe and supportive manner.

Patients with perinatal mental health conditions and OCD benefit from working with someone who has specialist expertise in managing these complex needs. Currently, in the NHS, the consensus is for a fixed number of sessions, typically short to medium term (six to twelve sessions). More research is needed in this area to establish the longevity and intensity of psychological treatment, as well as whether adjustments to the number and/or frequency of sessions affect the patient's clinical outcome and quality of life, based on measures in these areas.

Exposure and response prevention (ERP) therapy

Exposure and response prevention (ERP) is a special form of cognitive behavioural therapy that is used exclusively for the treatment of OCD. In ERP, not only are core beliefs scrutinised and intrusive thoughts challenged, but fears are faced head-on. ERP differs from CBT by placing the patient into an actual situation that causes them anxiety and distress while being encouraged to stay with the negative emotions until they subside. The more exposure, the better the response in terms of both the time required to come back to a neutral state and the degree of intensity they sustained from feared stimuli. In ERP, the therapist and patient work together to gradually expose the patient to their biggest fear. Like hiking up a mountain, the fears are tackled one step at a time, in a logical order.

Given the challenging and confrontational nature of ERP, it is unsurprising that it has a significant dropout rate. Nevertheless, this therapy alongside CBT for OCD is considered the gold standard for treatment. If it can be tolerated with the support of a specialist therapist trained in ERP techniques, it provides excellent outcomes in treating OCD (NICE 2005).

Concerns for the perinatal period

In clinical practice, there are two major concerns for accessing psychological therapy during the perinatal period. The first is readiness, both in terms of the patient's current situational factors (e.g. their imminent due date) and longer-term 'psychological mindedness', meaning their ability to understand, reflect, and engage with therapy. With CBT and ERP therapies, the patient must be willing and motivated to engage in their therapeutic process actively; not simply talking about their hopes and fears but physically confronting their worst thoughts and tolerating their subsequent feelings of distress. Even the most motivated individuals with support struggle with this, which may manifest in missing or cancelling appointments.

Another issue concerns the practicalities of childcare. Most services in the UK are not designed with baby in mind. Therapies such as CBT and ERP involve the patient and therapist alone. Specialist perinatal mental health services, however, often encourage babies into the therapy room, and some talking therapies in primary care offer childcare facilities onsite to allow patients to focus on therapy. Some may find it helpful to have baby in the room (e.g. fears involving harm to the child); for others, it may be too distracting, and childcare support will need to be arranged on a regular basis for treatment to continue.

Success in treatment will be very individual and based on the patient's main concerns. For all therapists, it's worthwhile to consider that living with uncertainty is one of the ultimate goals for the patient. This is especially true for patients in the perinatal period, particularly for those mothers with OCD and/or associated perfectionistic tendencies who struggle with this concept and loss of control. Being able to tolerate the not knowing and allowing life to unfold naturally may be one of the steepest therapeutic learning curves of all.

Flooding

For our honeymoon, I booked us into a beautiful, eco-friendly resort on a Malaysian island. We used an online travel agent who omitted a crucial detail: it was not just a luxury hotel but also a cat sanctuary for injured and neglected cats. While many would see this as a perk, I have a paralysing phobia of cats (known as ailurophobia, a term that I discovered while researching this book). I spent most of my honeymoon in terror among 50 cats, waking up with a cat on the bed or watching me sleep.

Over time, with support from my husband, I kept my composure around resort cats and managed to gently stroke a house cat on our last day. Although I still have a cat phobia, it's less severe now as I've slowly become familiar with calm cats of trusted friends.

I share this story as it is probably the best example I have personally of experiencing 'flooding', a version of exposure and response prevention that became more popular in the 1970s and 1980s, along with a 'facing your fears' and 'Frankie says relax' mindset. Much like someone learning to swim being thrown into the deep end on their first lesson, the theory behind flooding is to literally 'flood' the patient with so much exposure to their anxiety that they have no choice but to overcome the panic and face their fear head-on, hoping a survival instinct kicks in. Although some found this 'tough love' approach beneficial to some degree, most people found it not only terrifying but traumatising. Flooding would destroy not only the therapeutic trust but also any chance of recovery. Thankfully, exposure and response prevention has moved on considerably and is no longer using such cruel techniques to bring about change.

ART THERAPY

The current NICE guidelines for OCD/BDD and antenatal and postnatal mental health (NICE 2005) do not include art therapy. However, in clinical practice, the perinatal period is a prime time to explore the positive effects of arts and wellbeing on maternal mental health. The creative arts can be incorporated into wellbeing and recovery in a variety of ways through music, dance, and visual arts, for example. In this section, I use the example of creating a sewing group for women with perinatal OCD. Of course, one could replace the type of artistic project involved with another creative arts group, but the same principles (and challenges) will apply.

Examples of arts activities that could improve mental wellbeing include (as well as sewing) music groups, exercise groups, yoga, gardening, drawing, painting, singing groups, and mother and baby classes. Throughout my career, I have sought out those who have made positive and innovative change by including arts as part of their recovery process in mental health, maternity, and the criminal justice system, some of which are summarised in a report from the All-Party Parliamentary Group on Arts, Health and Wellbeing (2017). Another benefit of focusing on a creative activity (such as quilting, gardening, or drawing) is that it does not rely on using language and so is naturally inclusive of non-verbal communication for therapy. It also opens up the possibility of a therapeutic intervention that does not rely on the ability of an individual or group to disclose personal information if they do not feel ready to expose their vulnerability.

One powerful creative arts outlet is through the practice of sewing and quilting. Quilts have the power to not only bring people together, but also to connect generations and provide fuel for action against social injustice. In research into the benefits of quilting on wellbeing, Burt and Atkinson (2012) discovered several key themes, including positive aspects of creativity and control, social elements, and the finished product being tangible and purposeful. To my knowledge, there have been no specific studies looking into the use of creative arts for those with perinatal OCD. However, in the box below, I have described a few techniques from my own quilting practice that can be used to tackle perinatal OCD.

Creating a thoughtfully imperfect quilt: Helpful tips for those with OCD and perfectionism

During any arts-based project, someone with perfectionistic traits and perinatal OCD could become paralysed by their need for perfection, not feeling worthy to complete what's being made and use it. Finishing a quilt may also be problematic for those who struggle with order and symmetry, as they may choose to feed into this tendency by creating repetitive patterns within their work, re-measuring and re-arranging patchworks or making sure the points are perfectly aligned.

One way to tackle this is to encourage imperfection whilst quilting – what I like to call 'making mistakes on purpose'. This approach is adapted from ERP theory. I have done this in sewing workshops by simply reversing one of the pieced panels of the quilt and stitching the wrong side in place. This may initially increase anxiety in affected individuals, but encouraging them to sit with the emotion and continue with completing the project has therapeutic benefits. They can learn that their work of art is still beautiful, useful, and valid, even with its 'mistake'. If this is intolerable, and it may be, one can trial smaller and less noticeable errors on the back of the quilt (a side rarely seen) or ones that are so minor that only the quilter will ever notice. These include using a 'wrong' colour thread, stitching outside the line, or placing a quilt label inside out.

Another way to manage perfectionism or obsessions around symmetry is to refrain from the use of measuring tools and rulers by creating freehand, improvised quilts. These can be made using scraps of fabrics and quilting without a pattern. This encourages personal creative energy and improves confidence in one's ability to go off script and create something new and useful.

Finally, I would encourage participants to create something that would benefit or be useful to their baby, either while they're a baby or as an heirloom piece that can be passed down through generations. Not only will this give a wonderful emotive element to the project, but it has the potential to fill the individual with feelings of pride to see their child enjoying something that they have worked hard to complete. This can help balance the anxieties that may have cropped up during the creating process. Another option is for the individual to contribute to a group piece or pieces that can either be shared within the group or donated. This not only allows for creating a bigger piece or multiple smaller pieces in a short time frame but also allows for collaboration and communication between individuals towards a common shared goal, which may itself be therapeutic, as well as giving rise to the altruistic feelings involved in supporting others less fortunate than themselves. A good example of this is the London Modern Quilt Guild, who annually make quilted Christmas stockings for babies and their families admitted to the neonatal unit at the Evelina Children's Hospital in London.

PARENT–INFANT INTERVENTIONS

A key aspect in becoming a parent is establishing baby's emotional safety. If invested in from the beginning, emotional safety will transcend into building the internal sense of security and an inner world within the child that promotes self-esteem, self-confidence, and self-awareness.

Day-to-day activities between a parent and infant (such as feeding, playing, teasing, bathing) all help to build a predictable routine, which allows the child to feel safe and secure. However, it is not just the functional aspects of caregiving that are important. One must be engaged on a deeper, emotional level. Babies can pick up on the most subtle of cues; eye contact, smiling, hugging, soothing, acknowledgement, and mirroring all help to promote emotional wellbeing and a deep sense of security in themselves and the relationship. When mothers struggle with severe mental health issues, they may be distracted by their own thoughts (in perinatal OCD, obsessional thoughts and compulsive rituals). This distraction coupled with high stress and anxiety can have an effect on the bonding and attachment with their baby. This leads to insecure and preoccupied attachment styles later in life.

Perinatal mental health services and family wellbeing settings offer a unique form of therapy which involves assessment, observation, and an understanding of the parent–infant relationship, through parent–infant psychotherapy (PIP), video interactive guidance (VIG) therapy, or video interactive for positive parenting (VIPP) therapy. In recent years, these modalities of parent–infant focused screening tools, observations, and interventions have become more popular, from longer-term parent–infant psychotherapy to shorter periods of care through innovative video recording.

In Table 16.1, I summarise some adjunctive therapies that may be a useful tool in managing perinatal OCD. These are also useful for a whole host of other mental health conditions, including postnatal depression, anxiety, and personality disorder. The benefits of these newer methods include:

- they are non-invasive
- they can be used alongside or instead of medication
- they can provide lifelong skills whilst providing short-term impact and relief.

These methods focus on treating the parent as the expert on their baby, improving their own sense of self-esteem and parenting confidence. Specialist training in all these methods is available across the UK through the NHS. They are particularly aimed at those working in perinatal mental health, health visiting, and nursery settings.

Table 16.1 Adjunctive therapies in the perinatal period

Therapy	Description
Eye movement desensitisation and reprocessing (EMDR) therapy	A structured psychotherapy designed to help relieve stress from traumatic memories. Used predominantly in post-traumatic stress disorder but can also be used in other circumstances, such as tokophobia, panic disorder, and anxiety disorders.
Video-based interventions: video interactive guidance (VIG)/video interactive positive parenting (VIPP)	A strengths-based brief intervention where caregivers can watch recordings of their one-to-one interactions with their baby and then reflect with the therapist on their parenting and relationships. Utilises elements of parent–infant psychotherapy.
Compassion-focused therapy (CFT)	A structured psychological therapy that is supportive for those struggling with shame, self-criticism, and perfectionism. Utilises a combination of mindfulness techniques and cognitive behavioural techniques.
Schema-focused therapy	An integrative psychotherapy addressing early maladaptive schemas (unmet needs). Often rooted in childhood attachments such as feelings of abandonment, rejection, or over-vigilance.
Parent–infant psychotherapy	A longer-term psychotherapy focused on the parent–infant relationship. Often explores the experience of being parented/family relationships.
Art therapy/music therapy/drama therapy	A form of psychotherapy utilising the creative arts, such as drawing, painting, sculpting, music, or dance, to process emotions. Particularly useful for those who may struggle to verbalise their feelings.
Mindfulness-based interventions	Includes meditation, breathwork, mindfulness, and yoga to reduce stress and anxiety and to improve focus.
Systemic psychotherapy: couples therapy or family therapy	An intervention to help couples and/or families improve communication, resolve conflicts, and strengthen relationships.
Psychosexual therapy	Psychological intervention to help individuals/couples address sexual difficulties and/or sexual dysfunction.

Understanding the family script

Turning Red is a multicultural coming of age story released by Pixar in 2022. The story follows the plight of 13-year-old Canadian Chinese Mei Lee, who accidentally discovers an ancient generational gift (or curse by modern standards) whereby she turns into a large red panda when experiencing heightened emotions. This film, set against the backdrop of diverse Toronto, has been critically acclaimed as not just a nod to more representation in animation of both women and ethnic minorities, but also for the way it tackles, head-on, the skill of emotional intelligence and the intricacies of the mother–daughter relationship.

The film shines a light on the hidden pressures placed on children of first-generation migrant families to strive for excellence, not just academically, but socially as an all-round exemplar citizen representing their family, culture, and community. Mei Lee is torn between two worlds, the one of her mother's high expectations of her and the other (familiar to most teenage girls) of 'BFFs' and infatuation with boybands. Mei Lee's mother is depicted as an uptight parent who clearly loves her only child, but verges on being overbearing. This is done in a comical fashion, as she is seen hiding in the bushes with binoculars, watching Mei Lee when she is at school (to the point her friends begin to tease her about her 'control freak' mother), and being chased off school property by security.

When Mei Lee is taught the familial gift of the red panda, she learns that her mother also became a panda in her youth, as did all the mothers before her. We learn that Mei Lee's mother had a fraught relationship with her own mother as a teenager, and that she carried this tension to her mothering of her daughter. In her mind, she was doing all she could do to protect Mei Lee, while, in fact, she was stifling her, not allowing her to grow at her own pace and in her own time, let alone make any decisions for herself.

This story beautifully portrays the systemic concept of the familial script, a concept coined by pioneering family therapist John Byng-Hall in 1985. In essence, it describes how families often narrate stories about their lives, which they then pass down to their children. The way these stories are told (and, indeed, the stories that are untold due to shame and secrecy) colours our view of the world. For many, the story pattern is recycled generation after generation without a second thought. An example of a family script for Mei Lee is that the women in her family are strong and independent, and that emotions (depicted by the red panda) are a sign of shame and weakness. Mei Lee, however, finds the courage to not only question her mother, but her whole family belief system around striving for perfection. By the end of the movie (spoiler alert) she makes peace with her messy emotional side. Her father, who hilariously is allowed to speak very little, concludes the story with the poignant and affirming 'I love all sides of you.'

CHILDREN ARE THE FUTURE: PERINATAL MENTAL HEALTH, FAMILY THERAPY, AND THE EARLY YEARS

Although it is not recognised in the NICE guidelines for OCD, family therapy is recognised as pivotal in child and adolescent mental health, eating disorders, and more recently, perinatal mental health services. Family therapy not only addresses the individual's needs but also respects the 'space between people' in the interrelationships within the family. Family life can be complicated, and different relationships can exist between a mother and their son or daughter, as well as between the parents and siblings. Family relationships can become even more tangled when you consider the impact of grandparents, extended families, blended families, and the challenges family systems face when one member is unwell or when someone has passed away.

The family, of course, does not live in isolation, but is impacted by a whole host of external influences, such as school life, faith practices, and family ethnic identity, stories of migration, and feelings of belonging. Family therapy works by inviting a family to a series of therapy sessions. Usually, the family is observed in a clinical room with a two-way mirror. Behind this mirror is a team of trained family therapists. Tools may be used to facilitate discussions, such as positioning of stones or drawings, particularly if children are a part of the family work. After a period of observation, the therapists join the family and facilitate a discussion about the family dynamics and pertinent concerns presenting.

Although on the surface this may seem quite scary or non-traditional (compared with the idea of a patient and therapist alone in a room), the revelations can be quite amazing, providing a better understanding of family members and increased empathy. Importantly, the therapy can work even if a family member chooses to not attend, utilising the concept that even in absence, someone is making their presence known. Couples-focused therapy, alongside conventional treatments for OCD, may be helpful in circumstances where constant doubts continue to plague the relationship; it is accessible from most perinatal and/or primary care psychology NHS services.

There are many systemic psychotherapy approaches that can be adopted in the clinical setting outside formal therapy sessions. Below are two tools that I learned through my own systemic psychotherapy training and during my time working at the National OCD/BDD Unit that I use in my practice.

- *Drawing a family tree*: As an information-gathering exercise, particularly at the time of the initial assessment, I ask about personal and social history, trying to get a sense of the person's identity and experiences from childhood. I always draw a family tree, like those seen in genealogy work or the popular *Who Do You Think You Are?* documentary series on BBC that explores individual family history. In clinical settings, I add information about the names of family members and their relationships to the patient, which acts as a springboard for discussions about interfamilial relationships, as well as the history of mental illness within the family.

- *Externalising OCD*: Another technique I use, particularly in couple relationships entrenched in OCD behaviours, is that of 'You, me, and OCD'. Often in OCD, the illness can become so invasive it interferes with every part of the couple's life, including personal relationships. When living with someone with OCD, it can be hard to separate them from the illness. I ask couples to imagine that the OCD illness is their own person. They can even give it a name. During the session one can even pull up an empty chair for them, placed in between the couple for visual effect. I then suggest the couple talk to this person, placing all their anger, resentment, and worries onto this 'other' person. This not only serves to relieve the patient of the associated burden of carrying a mental illness but provides a hopeful place of restoration between the couple to understand that the illness is not synonymous with their identity; they can and do exist in their own right without the label or pain of perinatal mental illness and OCD. Similarly, intrusive unwanted thoughts can be given a name to separate them from one's true beliefs.

Looking to the future

In June 2021, the Princess of Wales launched the Royal Foundation Centre for Early Childhood, promoting research and collaboration of services to improve care for families while creating change by improving awareness and inspiring action to address the impact that the period from pregnancy to five years old has on adult life and future relationships (Royal Foundation n.d.). We are honoured to have leading figures in perinatal and infant mental health appointed as expert advisers to the centre, working alongside Her Royal Highness to shape the direction of children's and families' wellbeing, starting with much-needed work in the perinatal period.

Looking ahead, NHS England's long-term plan (Department of Health and Social Care 2025a), alongside the Royal College of Psychiatrists (2023a) report on infant and early childhood mental health, demonstrates a strong commitment to ensuring that perinatal mental health services continue to support not only women but also partners, children, and families. Beginning in the early years, the integration of parent–infant interventions with children and adolescent mental health services underscores the significance of emotional and psychological wellbeing from the outset of life. Further emphasis has been placed on a societal approach involving local communities, schools, and charitable sector organisations in supporting young families. This innovative practice has the potential to be life-changing for the future management and treatment of OCD, as many adults report experiencing their first symptoms during childhood. If addressed in the early years, there is hope of preventing the diagnosis from spiralling into adulthood and affecting their own parenting.

PHARMACOLOGICAL TREATMENT IN PREGNANCY AND BREASTFEEDING

The question I get asked the most frequently by patients in clinics (and colleagues in hospital corridors) is *'What is the best and safest medication to use in pregnancy and breastfeeding?'* The short answer is 'none'. That said, my perinatal colleagues and I do gravitate to certain medications that both our clinical experience and current evidence suggest work and that many patients find beneficial for alleviating their symptoms. However, several factors should be considered when deciding on pharmacological treatment.

We have known for many years that medication is effective in the treatment of OCD, either as an alternative to or in combination with psychological therapy for moderate-to-severe OCD. There is, however, a reluctance (or perhaps I should say a lack of understanding) regarding the pharmacological treatment options for anxiety disorders in general, with many professionals under the impression that management is 'purely psychological'. This belief does a disservice to patients who may feel stuck if they are not improving through talking therapy alone.

In this section, I hope to dispel myths surrounding medication use, particularly medication use for OCD in the perinatal period. I have also included a table summarising the common medications prescribed in the treatment of OCD (Table 16.2). The table includes information about the drugs and considerations for use during pregnancy and breastfeeding.

All drugs transfer to the placenta during pregnancy and to human milk in the postnatal period. The placenta, a new organ that develops as the baby grows, is responsible for retrieving nutrients and filtering out toxins that may harm the baby. While it is essential to be mindful of medication side effects, most medicines used to treat OCD and mental health conditions are safe for the unborn child. However, many women, particularly those who are anxious or concerned about potential harm to the baby, are hesitant to take medication, even when the risks are minimal. Those with OCD may also fixate on the particulars of medicines, the side effects profile, and the relative risks of every known adverse event, which only perpetuates the vicious cycle of OCD.

Using the RID score to assess risk

A well-recognised method for estimating risk during breastfeeding is to determine the relative infant dose (RID). The RID is calculated by dividing the infant's dose via milk (mg/kg/day) by the mother's dose (mg/kg/day). The score gives the clinician a guide for how much medication an infant may be exposed to on a weight-normalised basis (Hale 2021). Medications with a shorter half-life are preferred, as they generally reach their peak level and are eliminated from breast milk quickly. Some studies have indicated that discarding breast milk expressed when the peak level would be expected (four to five hours post-dose for most antidepressants) to be beneficial in reducing the overall bioavailability to the infant (Taylor, Barnes, & Young 2018).

Most herbal remedies, including vitamins and supplements, are not advised for use whilst breastfeeding due to the lack of evidence available and case reports of poisonous levels being found in newborns in contrast to during pregnancy (Guala et al. 2022). There are no regulatory guidelines nationally or internationally for an acceptable drug exposure for nursed children. However, it is widely accepted that an RID below 10% is considered compatible with breastfeeding. Most antidepressants have an RID below 5%. This does not include certain drugs that act on the central nervous system, which, due to their unique blood–brain barrier properties, may have a higher RID (up to 10%) yet remain well within safe limits. Barbiturates, benzodiazepines, and fluoxetine are specific examples where higher levels in the infant can occur due to their active metabolites. These may have a long paediatric half-life and accumulate in infant plasma over time. Thus, it is preferable to avoid them (Joint Formulary Committee 2024).

Challenges

Despite the documented benefits of breastfeeding, there is global concern regarding its uptake. The UK has the lowest rates in Europe (UNICEF UK n.d.). Several reasons contribute to why women cannot and/or choose not to breastfeed. In clinical practice, we recognise that a significant number of women with mental health difficulties opt not to breastfeed and/or discontinue breastfeeding prematurely due to the conflict they experience between breastfeeding and continuing prescribed medication, believing they must choose between breastfeeding and taking medication.

Many clinicians feel a lack of confidence in advising on best practice around medication use during breastfeeding or, being overcautious, advise not to breastfeed as a safe bet. Evidence shows that most mothers can continue to breastfeed and take prescribed medication without risk to the child.

Although we know the temptation for a rapid, binary answer in clinical settings to whether a medication is safe to continue, the reality informing an answer is often more complex. It requires an in-depth assessment, preferably with referral to a perinatal psychiatrist. These specialist clinicians will often welcome a referral. They have the medical expertise to understand medication use for those breastfeeding, are regularly updated with the latest evidence-based guidance on medication use, and can provide a biopsychosocial approach to treatment options, along with a risk–benefit analysis for the mother (medical and psychiatric risk) and infant in the postnatal period.

What to prescribe

Antidepressants are the drug of choice, specifically SSRIs (selective serotonin reuptake inhibiters). These drugs were developed in the 1970s and work on the chemical pathways in the brain, in a complex way but ultimately allowing more of the 'happy hormone' serotonin to be readily available. Examples of SSRIs we routinely use in clinical practice include citalopram, escitalopram, paroxetine, and fluoxetine. Each patient is unique, and some may respond well to one drug but not another. Even within the same SSRI family of medications, there may be some trial and error in choosing the best medication. However, one should try to limit exposure to two or more antidepressants during development *in utero*.

Similarly, each SSRI has unique properties and cautions to be mindful of when prescribing in pregnancy. The risks and benefits need to be weighed and discussed with the patient when considering treatment. NICE guidelines in antenatal mental health recommend that when a mother takes medication for treatment for mental health prior to conceiving, it is best to continue with that medication through pregnancy and not to 'stop and change' just because she is pregnant (Stahl 2020).

Clomipramine is another type of antidepressant (a tricyclic antidepressant or TCA), which has unique properties that are found to be useful in OCD treatment and more effective than other TCAs (Del Casale et al. 2019). One must, however, be cautious in using a tricyclic antidepressant with those that have a history of self-harm or suicide attempts. Medication overdose is lethal in this subgroup, as clomipramine and other TCAs can affect the QTc interval (related to heart rate), resulting in severe cardiac toxicity. This could lead to intensive-care support and even death following overdose (Sharma 2018).

Table 16.2 summarises the antidepressants commonly used to treat OCD. It includes dosage recommendations, class of medication, mechanism of action, and considerations for use in pregnancy (by trimester) and breastfeeding. This summary is merely a guide. Any clinical decision needs to be made on a case-by-case basis in collaboration with the patient. When considering prescribing medication in the perinatal period, one must have an open and transparent discussion about the benefits and known risks associated with medication use during pregnancy (which may vary depending on the trimester) and while breastfeeding. This enables the patient to make an informed decision about commencing treatment.

Treatment success

Combining medication with psychological therapy (either together or consecutively) has been shown to be more beneficial than either approach alone (Nezgovorova et al. 2022). Determining treatment 'success' has largely been subjective; however, it can be measured in several ways, such as reduction in symptoms, as noted by repeating the OCD screening questionnaire before and after treatment, or additional questionnaires assessing how much individuals feel they have improved. Objective improvement may also be observed in the patient's interactions with others, enhanced attachment and bonding with their baby, and increased ability to engage in daily living activities with a reduction in time spent on such activities (including obsessional ruminations).

Table 16.2 Antidepressants in pregnancy and breastfeeding

Drug	Mechanism	Dose	Pregnancy	Breastfeeding	Common side effects
Sertraline	SSRI	50–200mg	Safe and recommended in pregnancy Monitor for neonatal discontinuation syndrome	Undetectable/trace amounts in breast milk (<1%) Not dose-dependent	Nausea and vomiting Reduced libido Sleep disturbance Headache
Citalopram	SSRI	20–40mg	Safe and recommended in pregnancy Monitor for neonatal discontinuation syndrome	Advised to continue if used in pregnancy Approx. 0–5% detected in breast milk Dose-dependent	Nausea and vomiting Reduced libido Sleep disturbance Headache
Escitalopram	SSRI	10–20mg	Safe and recommended in pregnancy Monitor for neonatal discontinuation syndrome	Advised to continue if used in pregnancy Approx. 0–8% detected in breast milk Dose-dependent	Nausea and vomiting Reduced libido Sleep disturbance Headache
Fluoxetine	SSRI	20–80mg	Safe and recommended in pregnancy Monitor for neonatal discontinuation syndrome	Advised to continue if used in pregnancy Breakdown product norfluoxetine, higher levels (approx. 3–12%) detected in breast milk Monitor for colic, agitation, irritability, poor feeding, and poor weight gain in newborn	Nausea and vomiting Reduced libido Sleep disturbance Headache
Paroxetine	SSRI	20–60mg	Small increased risk of CV malformations in first trimester Monitor for neonatal discontinuation syndrome	Relatively safe to use Approx. 1–5% detected in breast milk	Nausea and vomiting Reduced libido Sleep disturbance Headache Drowsiness
Clomipramine	TCA	100–200mg	Small increased risk of CV malformations in first trimester Monitor for neonatal discontinuation syndrome	Relatively safe to use but limited studies Undetectable amounts in breast milk at doses <125mcg Approx. 1–2% concentration in breast milk at higher doses (>125mcg)	Blurred vision Constipation Dry mouth Sedation Increased appetite

One must also be mindful of the time span for defining success. In an ideal world, success would equate to total remission and cure of the illness. We are fortunate that OCD, compared to every other mental illness, is a highly treatable condition and many have been cured of this disorder after a period of targeted treatment of psychological therapy in combination with medication use.

However, we know that OCD is often under-reported, under-detected and under-diagnosed, thus barriers to treatment success are created even before setting foot in the therapist's room. For those receiving treatment, the dose of medication and/or number of psychological sessions may not be optimal, often leaving patients dissatisfied, feeling 'only half-better'. OCD is also unique in that in partially treated or untreated patients (or even in those who feel they have fully recovered) symptoms can resurface and may morph into different themes, reflective of the different stages in their life (e.g. previously being worried about contamination fears before having a baby, and then later becoming preoccupied with harm coming to their child).

Success may be seen after one, three, or six months of treatment. One might argue that the goal is to reassess at longer intervals (one to five years) to see whether the treatment has longevity. This might be possible now that perinatal services in the UK are slowly changing to reflect the government's drive towards improving services for young people, with greater emphasis on 0–5-year-olds and family mental wellbeing (Royal College of Psychiatrists 2023a).

When using medication to treat OCD, symptomatic improvement is seen at the maximum dosage (aka, titration to the highest dose available). For example, if prescribing sertraline, one would expect a breakthrough in improvement when dosing reaches 150mg or 200mg once daily, if tolerated. This is important, as many patients are prescribed antidepressants in primary care but are often left on the lowest dose (50mg once a day) without further review or increase, noting limited symptomatic relief and only a partial response to treatment. Sadly, many discontinue the medication, feeling it is not working.

When explaining this dilemma in clinic, I liken it to having the worst migraine but only taking half a paracetamol tablet to cure it. Such a tiny dose won't touch excruciating pain associated with migraines and their auras. It is important, then, to treat the condition with not only the correct medication but also at the right dosage.

Should an SSRI medication at its highest dose in combination with psychological/behavioural intervention still not provide symptomatic relief, one might, in severe cases, consider adding (augmenting) another drug to boost the effects of the antidepressant medication. Traditionally, low-dose antipsychotic medication has been used. Some OCD studies suggest moderate improvements when an SSRI is combined with either olanzapine, lamotrigine, risperidone, or quetiapine (Maiti et al. 2023; Thamby & Jaisoorya 2019).

However, we are mindful that our patients who are either pregnant and/or breastfeeding have special considerations separate from the general OCD population. Risperidone, for example, is not advised for use in pregnant or lactating women, as one of the side effects is the interruption of prolactin production, which can affect breastfeeding and fertility (Betcher, Montiel, & Clark 2019). Newer studies on OCD augmentation and clinical practice use aripiprazole, a dopamine partial agonist, which also has serotonergic properties, and relatively few side effects compared to other antipsychotics (Albert et al. 2018; Cuomo, Goracci, & Fagiolini 2018; Tosato et al. 2017). It is one of the few psychotropic medications that does not have a causal link with weight gain, so may be particularly advantageous to women during the perinatal period if they are at risk of obstetric complications due to higher BMI, or have metabolic conditions such as gestational diabetes (NICE 2005, 2014)

Factors influencing medication choice

It is not only the medication's side effects that influence the decision of choosing medication; other factors include:

- the patient's preferences
- past medication history (including previous experience of side effects)
- comorbid medical conditions
- comorbid psychiatric conditions
- whether pregnant or postnatal
- whether choosing to breastfeed or mix formula and breastfeed

- historical responsiveness to psychological/pharmacological interventions
- individual/cultural attitudes towards medication use in general.

Given the multiple complexities to consider when prescribing treatment for OCD in the perinatal period, research recommends referral in the first instance to a specialist perinatal psychiatrist to review, commence and monitor medication use and symptomatic response (Sharma 2018). If available, I would also recommend discussing the latest evidence-based research with a specialist perinatal pharmacist or teratology information service.

Medications and neuroplasticity

Currently, there is some exciting research in the field of treating OCD, linking traditional psychotherapy with new advances in neuroplasticity (Faustino 2022). This research is based on the understanding that neurones in the brain are not fixed but can adapt, change, and even form new connections. D-cycloserine, an N-methyl-D-aspartic (NMDA) agonist, has been shown in preliminary studies to eradicate fear in both rats and humans and, when administered in short bursts, can enhance responsiveness to psychological therapies (although it does not necessarily alleviate overall symptoms of OCD).

Similarly, there is renewed interest in using psychedelic drugs to treat mental health disorders. Psychedelics were studied in the 1960s, with hallucinogens like LSD used as adjuncts in psychotherapy to help patients 'open up', leading to consideration of combined drug and psychotherapeutic treatments (Tolin & Worden 2012). Recently, a landmark study was published exploring the efficacy and mechanisms of psilocybin, a serotonin receptor agonist, for treating OCD in adults (Pellegrini et al. 2025). The results are promising; however, there are still several gaps in our knowledge regarding the treatment of perinatal OCD.

More research is needed

As we've discussed earlier, our ability to incorporate the latest research in the perinatal population is still growing, but it faces some challenges. Ethical concerns about involving pregnant and breastfeeding women in clinical trials – since there could be unknown risks to the baby during pregnancy or through milk – play a big part. It's important to keep in mind that any advice we give is based on the current knowledge and may not be applicable in the future. When it comes to medication use for treating perinatal OCD, we're still in the early stages of understanding, and new discoveries could lead to changes in guidance down the line. We look forward to more research helping us provide safer, more effective care over time.

CHAPTER 17

The Past, Present, and Future of Perinatal OCD Treatment

NEUROSURGERY AND NEUROMODULATION

Around Freud's psychoanalytical era, brain dissection gained popularity as a treatment for severe mental illness, serving as a mid-century alternative to asylums (Lapidus et al. 2013). Psychosurgery was historically used for OCD and other psychiatric conditions, but early 20th-century procedures were seen as crude and barbaric. Lobectomies, involving the removal of brain lobes, were common yet comparable to amputating a hand for a broken nail. These operations, often called experiments, targeted marginalised individuals, including women with little choice but to trust their doctors (Tone & Koziol 2018). This treatment method, alongside electroconvulsive therapy, remains stigmatised, evoking images of *Frankenstein* and *One Flew Over the Cuckoo's Nest*, with health professionals portrayed as the 'Mad Professor' or 'Nurse Ratchet'.

The landscape of OCD treatment options is changing quickly. In particular, invasive and non-invasive methods involving brain stimulation and manipulation have been controversial but highly anticipated. Currently, neurosurgery is not recommended for OCD treatment within the NHS in the UK. However, there is a subgroup with severe impairment and treatment resistance for whom neurosurgery – specifically anterior cingulotomy or capsulotomy – may be an option. If considered necessary in extreme cases, this option must be discussed and arranged through a specialist OCD service and must meet the criteria for neurosurgery, including strict ethical protocols (NICE 2005, 2021).

The use of neuromodulation techniques, such as deep brain stimulation (DBS), as a treatment for OCD has been introduced as an alternative to neurosurgical ablation for various reasons, particularly because it is reversible and adjustable at the sites of the ventral capsule and ventral striatum in the forebrain (Tyagi et al. 2019). The next sections discuss DBS and transcranial magnetic stimulation (TMS), and while neither is currently available for clinical treatment on the NHS, they can be accessed through the private sector and in research settings. These newer technologies hold significant promise in other areas of mental health research. In theory, they may be preferred during the perinatal period, as they are non-invasive and pose minimal risk during pregnancy or breastfeeding; however, more research is urgently needed in this area to facilitate dissemination into clinical practice. Both could be life-changing, as they enable management and treatment of severe mental illness during pregnancy and the postnatal period, potentially in an outpatient or day hospital setting, with minimal pre-operative and post-operative monitoring.

Practical factors (such as childcare and separation from the baby) and risks to the foetus are often among the biggest hurdles women face when seeking treatment during the perinatal period. These non-invasive, specialist, and focused brain treatments could address these issues, offering new hope for the future of treating severe perinatal OCD.

DEEP BRAIN STIMULATION

In 2009, deep brain stimulation was approved in the US to treat patients with severe OCD who had been unresponsive to specialised CBT and medication. DBS is a neurosurgical technique that involves placing electrodes in the brain, which send an electrical current to target specific areas influencing psychiatric and neurological symptoms. The wires are externally attached to a pulse generator, which is usually fixed under the skin in the chest area, similar to a heart pacemaker.

Research indicates that applying DBS to the anterior limb of the internal area of the internal capsule, deep within the cerebral hemisphere, could improve OCD symptoms with only minimal side effects (Slepneva et al. 2024). Over time, with advancements in our understanding of neuroimaging and the pathways involved in severe OCD, clinicians are now able to identify additional areas of the brain that respond to OCD treatment. While the optimal target for OCD is still being refined, approximately 60% of patients undergoing DBS have shown significant and sustained reductions in both obsessions and compulsive behaviour. The success of DBS therapy for OCD has expanded the potential range of applications to other related psychiatric disorders such as Tourette syndrome and major depression. DBS also offers the advantage of being reversible in nature and carries a relatively small operative risk compared to traditional neurosurgery techniques (Aum & Tierney 2018; Rapinesi et al. 2019). Van Westen et al. (2015) note that DBS can objectively reduce symptom scale ratings post-procedure with up to 58% improvement and help individuals resume a good quality of life.

TRANSCRANIAL MAGNETIC STIMULATION

Transcranial magnetic stimulation (TMS) and transcranial direct-current stimulation (TDCS) are also non-invasive procedures growing in popularity for treatment of psychiatric and neurological disorders. In TMS treatment, a magnetic plate (similar to an MRI machine) is secured just above the scalp. This emits a magnetic field to a targeted area of the brain. The patient remains awake throughout the session, which usually takes approximately 20 to 30 minutes. By modulating excitatory and inhibitory areas of the brain, TMS aims to improve cognitive functioning, and has been experimented with in several conditions, including dementia, Parkinson's disease, depression, and epilepsy.

Like DBS, TMS is both adjustable and reversible, and it carries a lesser side effect burden compared to neurosurgical ablation. There is a growing body of research interest in its use as an alternative to medication, which may be advantageous in the perinatal period due to its non-invasive nature (e.g. Stengel et al. 2022; Yuvaci et al. 2019). It is regarded as a potential alternative to electroconvulsive therapy, which has been employed to treat women with severe antenatal and postnatal depression. Further research is required in this area, particularly regarding its potential benefits for the treatment of perinatal OCD (Begemann et al. 2020).

In conclusion, the future is bright. The UK is leading the way in terms of novel treatments for OCD, as well as the call for action to support the mental health of infants and children. There are several options available for the treatment of perinatal OCD, and these can be tailored to a variety of settings to suit the mother and baby. Referral into services to access this support, however, remains a complex issue, hindered by stigma and fear. My hope is that the guidance provided will equip health professionals and families with the additional understanding and skills to both offer reassurance and advocate for those that may find it hard to advocate for themselves when struggling with OCD during the transition to motherhood.

Epilogue

> ***Macbeth:*** *How does your patient, doctor?*
> ***Doctor:*** *Not so sick, my lord, as she is troubled with thick-coming fancies that keep her from rest.*
> ***Macbeth:*** *Cure her of that! Canst thou not minister to a mind diseased, pluck from the memory a rooted sorrow, raze out the written troubles of the brain, and with some sweet oblivious antidote cleanse the stuffed bosom of that perilous stuff which weighs upon her heart?*
> ***Doctor:*** *Therein the patient must minister to himself.*
>
> WILLIAM SHAKESPEARE, *THE TRAGEDY OF MACBETH*

Many scholars have analysed this famous scene from *The Tragedy of Macbeth*, as both Macbeth and his wife, Lady Macbeth, spiral into madness after committing high treason and murder. But what does this have to do with perinatal OCD and mental health? As a health professional – whether you are a midwife, social worker, GP, or therapist – you will at some point find yourself in the middle of a crisis in someone's life or helping others while experiencing personal crises of your own. Our patients seek help when they are in desperate need (and sometimes frustrated) to 'cure her of that!' This cure might involve a pill, therapy, or delivering the baby (or a combination of all three). When young children are involved and the mother, who is usually the primary caregiver, finds herself bedridden and broken, the stakes are even higher. Shakespeare reminds us 'the patient must minister to himself', implying that Macbeth must also address his inner ills if he is to support Lady Macbeth in making a full recovery.

Although this book primarily focuses on understanding and

treating perinatal OCD, it also provides another essential piece of the puzzle: the importance of looking after oneself, whether you are a clinician, carer, or both. As a healthcare professional, it is crucial to prioritise your own wellbeing, because if your emotional health is neglected, it becomes much more difficult to care for others. Being a therapist (and I use that term loosely to include anyone engaging with a patient) can take a toll on both body and mind. Burnout is common in the medical field, with more doctors taking time out of training and leaving the profession than ever before. In our psychiatry training, we are fortunate to have wellbeing taken seriously; we are one of the few medical specialities with mandatory weekly supervision for trainees, with a focus on reflective practice to process the daily challenges faced when caring for those with severe mental illness.

In midwifery, the situation is worse. Consider the undeniable stress placed on professionals entering maternity services, often young women of childbearing age. They are thrown into high-risk clinical situations, often a matter of life and death, with very little time for reflection or recovery. And I was shocked to learn that even my colleagues working in oncology, delivering news of the dreaded 'c-word', or those in the A&E trauma unit, have no regular supportive reflective groups or supervision. It is no wonder that doctors are the profession with the highest rates of alcohol abuse: drinking to process, or should I say numb, their emotions.

There are many ways to enhance emotional resilience and wellbeing, both of which are essential skills for working in healthcare services. Many self-help books have been written on this topic. However, this book focuses on the nature of OCD. The condition can manifest in various ways, and those living with or caring for someone with OCD can easily experience caregiver burnout. Constant reassurance-seeking can be challenging and exhausting, not only for the person seeking reassurance but also for the one providing it. OCD is also a condition where transference can occur, meaning that the patient's inner emotions can become mirrored in yourself. You may suddenly notice your anxiety increasing after spending time with someone with severe OCD. This is related to transference. Taking care of your emotional needs will help to reduce this. Healthy sleep habits, balanced nutrition, regular exercise (which boosts endorphins and relieves stress), and incorporating reflective practices into your day (such as journalling, prayer, meditation, etc.) are the foundational pillars of wellbeing.

Other important practices include:

- Staying connected: Meet with friends and family to relax in each other's company.

- ...but disconnect: Switch off your phone. Turn off notifications. Do not fall into the trap of replying to work emails late into the night.

- Finding your 'happy hobby': Discovering a new skill and taking up a hobby later in life can bring great joy and serve as a good activity to lean on during stressful moments.

- Taking breaks: Use your annual leave! You don't get a medal at the end of the year for not taking your leave. Your annual leave days are intended as protective buffers to prevent burnout and keep you from becoming physically and mentally exhausted. Try to travel if you can, as this will help you shift into relaxation and rejuvenation mode.

- Boundaries. Boundaries. Boundaries: Hold tight to your boundaries and protect them fiercely.

- Reflection and supervision: Regardless of your role, if you are caring for patients with OCD and/or other mental health needs, please seek out someone you trust for supervision to discuss cases, or join a group to reflect. This will significantly lessen the emotional burden on you and provide a much-needed outlet, so you don't end up 'taking your work home with you' (and shouting at the children/dog because of it).

References

Abramowitz, J.S., & Jacoby, R.J. (2014). Scrupulosity: A cognitive-behavioral analysis and implications for treatment. *Journal of Obsessive-Compulsive and Related Disorders*, *3*(1), 140–149.

Abramowitz, J.S., Meltzer-Brody, S., Leserman, J., Killenberg, S., et al. (2010). Obsessional thoughts and compulsive behaviours in a sample of women with postpartum mood symptoms. *Archives of Women's Mental Health*, *13*(6), 523–530.

Abramowitz, J.S., Schwartz, S.A., & Moore, K.M. (2003a). Obsessional thoughts in postpartum females and their partners: Content, severity, and relationship with depression. *Journal of Clinical Psychology in Medical Settings*, *10*, 157–164.

Abramowitz, J.S., Schwartz, S.A., Moore, K.M., & Luenzmann, K.R. (2003b). Obsessive-compulsive symptoms in pregnancy and the puerperium: A review of the literature. *Journal of Anxiety Disorders*, *17*, 461–478.

Agardh, C., Asamoah, B.O., Herder, T., & Larsson, M. (2022). Risk of poor mental health and experience of violence among a young adult population with same-sex sexuality: A cross-sectional study in southern Sweden. *BMJ Open*, *12*, e052617. doi:10.1136/bmjopen-2021-052617

Ahn, L.H., Keum, B.T., Meizys, G.M., Choudry, A., Gomes, M.A., & Wang, L. (2022). Second-generation Asian American women's gendered racial socialization. *Journal of Counseling Psychology*, *69*(2), 129–145.

Ainsworth, M.D., & Bell, S.M. (1970). Attachment, exploration, and separation: Illustrated by the behavior of one-year-olds in a strange situation. *Child Development*, *41*(1), 49–67.

Albert, U., Marazziti, D., Di Salvo, G., Solia, F., Rosso, G., & Maina, G. (2018). A systematic review of evidence-based treatment strategies for obsessive-compulsive disorder resistant to first-line pharmacotherapy. *Current Medicinal Chemistry*, *25*(41), 5647–5661.

All-Party Parliamentary Group on Arts, Health and Wellbeing (2017). *Creative Health: The Arts for Health and Wellbeing*. https://ncch.org.uk/uploads/Creative_Health_Inquiry_Report_2017_-_Second_Edition.pdf

Alonso, P., Menchón, J.M., Mataix-Cols, D., Pifarré, J., et al. (2004). Perceived parental rearing style in obsessive-compulsive disorder: Relation to symptom dimensions. *Psychiatry Research*, *127*(3), 267–278.

Ashraf, F., & Jepsen, D. (2024). Private patriarchy's impact on women's careers: Through kaleidoscope career model lens. *Group & Organization Management*, *0*(0). doi:10.1177/10596011241227263

Aum, D.J., & Tierney, T.S. (2018). Deep brain stimulation: Foundations and future trends. *Frontiers in Bioscience (Landmark Edition), 23*(1), 162–182.

Ayers, S., Bond, R., Bertullies, S., & Wijma, K. (2016). The aetiology of post-traumatic stress following childbirth: A meta-analysis and theoretical framework. *Psychological Medicine, 46*(6), 1121–1134.

Ayers, S., Eagle, A., & Waring, H. (2006). The effects of childbirth-related post-traumatic stress disorder on women and their relationships: A qualitative study. *Psychology, Health & Medicine, 11*(4), 389–398.

Bartholomew, M.K., Schoppe-Sullivan, S.J., Glassman, M., Kamp Dush, C.M., & Sullivan, J.M. (2012). New parents' Facebook use at the transition to parenthood. *Family Relations, 61*(3), 455–469.

Barton, R., Aouad, P., Hay, P., Buckett, G., et al. (2022). Distinguishing delusional beliefs from overvalued ideas in anorexia nervosa: An exploratory pilot study. *Journal of Eating Disorders, 10*(1), 85.

Bass, C., & Glaser, D. (2014). Early recognition and management of fabricated or induced illness in children. *Lancet, 383*(9926), 1412–1421.

Baumrind, D. (1966). Effects of authoritative parental control on child behaviour. *Child Development, 37*(4), 887–907.

Begemann, M.J., Brand, B.A., Ćurčić-Blake, B., Aleman, A., & Sommer, I.E. (2020). Efficacy of non-invasive brain stimulation on cognitive functioning in brain disorders: A meta-analysis. *Psychological Medicine, 50*(15), 2465–2486.

Beheshti, M., Rabiei, N., Taghizadieh, M., Eskandari, P., et al. (2023). Correlations between single nucleotide polymorphisms in obsessive-compulsive disorder with the clinical features or response to therapy. *Journal of Psychiatric Research, 157*, 223–238.

Berg, B. (2020, 6 October). Nobody know why this mother bear is so aggressive, but her fans love it. *The Guardian*. www.theguardian.com/environment/2020/oct/06/aggressive-mother-bear-alaska-fans-online

Berrios, G.E. (1989). Obsessive-compulsive disorder: Its conceptual history in France during the 19th century. *Comprehensive Psychiatry, 30*(4), 283–295.

Betancourt, H., & López, S.R. (1993). The study of culture, ethnicity, and race in American psychology. *American Psychologist, 48*(6), 629–637.

Betcher, H.K., Montiel, C., & Clark, C.T. (2019). Use of antipsychotic drugs during pregnancy. *Current Treatment Options in Psychiatry, 6*(1), 17–31.

Bezahler, A., Kuckertz, J.M., McKay, D., Falkenstein, M.J., & Feinstein, B.A. (2024). Emotion regulation and OCD among sexual minority people: Identifying treatment targets. *Journal of Anxiety Disorders, 101*, 102807. doi:10.1016/j.janxdis.2023.102807

Birth Trauma Association (n.d.). What is birth trauma? www.birthtraumaassociation.org/what-is-birth-trauma

Bloch, M.H., Landeros-Weisenberger, A., Sen, S., Dombrowski, P., et al. (2008). Association of the serotonin transporter polymorphism and obsessive-compulsive disorder: Systematic review. American *Journal of Medical Genetics B Neuropsychiatric Genetics, 147B*(6), 850–858.

Bodri, D., Nair, S., Gill, A., Lamanna, G., et al. (2018). Shared motherhood IVF: High delivery rates in a large study of treatments for lesbian couples using partner-donated eggs. *Reproductive Biomedicine Online, 36*(2), 130–136.

Bogousslavsky, J., & Dieguez, S. (2014). Sigmund Freud and hysteria: The etiology of psychoanalysis? *Frontiers of Neurology and Neuroscience, 35*, 109–125.

Bowlby, J. (1951). Maternal care and mental health. *Bulletin of the World Health Organization, 3*, 355–533.

Bradford, J.M. (1999). The paraphilias, obsessive compulsive spectrum disorder, and the treatment of sexually deviant behaviour. *Psychiatric Quarterly, 70*(3), 209–219.

Bradley, R., & Slade, P. (2011). A review of mental health problems in fathers following the birth of a child. *Journal of Reproductive and Infant Psychology, 29*(1), 19–42.

Brander, G., Rydell, M., Kuja-Halkola, R., de la Cruz, L.F., et al. (2016). Association of perinatal risk factors with obsessive-compulsive disorder: A population-based birth cohort, sibling control study. *JAMA Psychiatry, 73*(11), 1135–1144.

Brandes, M., Soares, C.N., & Cohen, L.S. (2004). Postpartum onset obsessive-compulsive disorder: Diagnosis and management. *Archives of Women's Mental Health, 7*(2), 99–110.

Bretherton, I. (1992). The origins of attachment theory: John Bowlby and Mary Ainsworth. *Developmental Psychology, 28*(5), 759–775.

Brewin, C.R., Atwoli, L., Bisson, J.I., Galea, S., Koenen, K., & Lewis-Fernández, R. (2025). Post-traumatic stress disorder: Evolving conceptualization and evidence, and future research directions. *World Psychiatry, 24*(1), 52–80.

Bridges, R.S. (2020). The behavioral neuroendocrinology of maternal behavior: Past accomplishments and future directions. *Hormones and Behavior, 120*, 104662. doi:10.1016/j.yhbeh.2019.104662

Brune, M. (2006). The evolutionary psychology of obsessive-compulsive disorder: The role of cognitive meta representation. *Perspectives in Biology and Medicine, 49*(3), 317–329.

Burt, E.L., & Atkinson, L. (2012). The relationship between quilting and wellbeing. *Journal of Public Health, 34*(1), 54–59.

Burton, H. (2021). How women with established obsessive compulsive disorder experience pregnancy and postpartum: An interpretative phenomenological analysis. *Journal of Reproductive and Infant Psychology, 39*(3), 313–325.

Byng-Hall, J. (1985). The family script: A useful bridge between theory and practice. *Journal of Family Therapy, 7*, 301–305.

Chaudhary, S., Singh, A.P., & Varshney, A. (2022). Psychodynamic perspective of sexual obsessions in obsessive-compulsive disorder. *Annals of Neurosciences, 29*(2–3), 159–165.

Chaudron, L.H., & Nirodi, N. (2010). The obsessive-compulsive spectrum in the perinatal period: A prospective pilot study. *Archives of Women's Mental Health, 13*, 5, 403–410.

Child Safeguarding Practice Review Panel (2021). *'The Myth of Invisible Men': Safeguarding Children under 1 from Non-accidental Injury Caused by Male Carers*. https://assets.publishing.service.gov.uk/government/uploads/system/uploads/attachment_data/file/1017944/The_myth_of_invisible_men_safeguarding_children_under_1_from_non-accidental_injury_caused_by_male_carers.pdf

Clark, S., & Coker, S. (2009). Perfectionism, self-criticism and maternal criticism: A study of mothers and their children. *Personality and Individual Differences, 47*(4), 321–325.

Cleghorn, E. (2021). *Unwell Women: Misdiagnosis and Myth in a Man-Made World*. Dutton.

Cohen, L., Maroun, M., & Wagner, S. (2018). Behavior: Oxytocin promotes fearless motherhood. *Current Biology*, *28*(8), R359–R361.

Conceição Costa, D.L., Chagas Assunção, M., Arzeno Ferrão, Y., Archetti Conrado, L., et al. (2012). Body dysmorphic disorder in patients with obsessive-compulsive disorder: Prevalence and clinical correlates. *Depression and Anxiety*, *29*(11), 966–975.

Cosh, S.M., Olson, J., & Tully, P.J. (2023). Exploration of orthorexia nervosa and diagnostic overlap with eating disorders, anorexia nervosa and obsessive-compulsive disorder. *International Journal of Eating Disorders*, *56*(11), 2155–2161.

Crittenden, P. (2005). Der CARE-Index als Hilfsmittel für Früherkennung, Intervention und Forschung [Using the CARE-Index for screening, intervention, and research]. Frühförderung Interdisziplinär [Early Interdisciplinary Intervention; Special issue]. *Bindungsorientierte Ansätze in der Praxis der Frühförderung*, *24*, S99–S106.

Cuomo, A., Goracci, A., & Fagiolini, A. (2018). Aripiprazole use during pregnancy, peripartum and lactation: A systematic literature search and review to inform clinical practice. *Journal of Affective Disorders*, *228*, 229–237.

de Beauvoir, S. (2015). *The Second Sex*. Vintage Classics. Original work published 1949.

Del Casale, A., Sorice, S., Padovano, A., Simmaco, M., et al. (2019). Psychopharmacological treatment of obsessive-compulsive disorder (OCD). *Current Neuropharmacology*, *17*(8), 710–736.

de Leon, J., Bott, A., & Simpson, G.M. (1989). Dysmorphophobia: Body dysmorphic disorder or delusional disorder, somatic subtype? *Comprehensive Psychiatry*, *30*(6), 457–472.

Department of Health (1998). *Working Together to Safeguard: New Government Proposals for Inter-Agency Cooperation*. Consultation Paper. London: DoH.

Department of Health and Social Care (2025a). *Fit for the Future: 10 Year Health Plan for England*. www.gov.uk/government/publications/10-year-health-plan-for-england-fit-for-the-future

Department of Health and Social Care (2025b). Improved safeguarding and protections for vulnerable people [Press release]. www.gov.uk/government/news/improved-safeguarding-and-protections-for-vulnerable-people

Dondu, A., Caliskan, M., & Orenay-Boyacioglu, S. (2022). Link between obsessive-compulsive disorder and polymorphisms in HDAC genes. *Brazilian Journal of Psychiatry*, *44*(2), 156–163.

Dorfan, N.M., & Woody, S.R. (2012). Assessing OCD Symptoms and Severity. In G. Steketee (Ed.) *The Oxford Handbook of Obsessive Compulsive and Spectrum Disorders* (pp.254–274). Oxford Academic.

Douglas, S., & Michaels, M. (2004). *The Mommy Myth: The Idealisation of Motherhood and How It Has Undermined Women*. Free Press.

Edwards, E., & Timmons, S. (2005). A qualitative study of stigma among women suffering postnatal illness. *Journal of Mental Health*, *14*(5), 471–481.

Esch, T., & Stefano, G.B. (2005). The neurobiology of love. *Neuro Endocrinology Letters*, *26*(3), 175–192.

Faden, J., Levin, J., Mistry, R., & Wang, J. (2017). Delusional disorder, erotomanic type, exacerbated by social media use. *Case Reports in Psychiatry*, 8652524. doi:10.1155/2017/8652524

Fairbrother, N., Collardeau, F., Albert, A.Y.K., Challacombe, F.L., et al. (2021). High prevalence and incidence of obsessive-compulsive disorder among women across pregnancy and the postpartum. *Journal of Clinical Psychiatry, 82*(2), 20m13398. doi:10.4088/JCP.20m13398

Faustino, B. (2022). Minding my brain: Fourteen neuroscience-based principles to enhance psychotherapy responsiveness. *Clinical Psychology & Psychotherapy, 29*(4), 1254–1275.

Feng, L., Zhang, L., & Zhong, H. (2021). Perceived parenting styles and mental health: The multiple mediation effect of perfectionism and altruistic behavior. *Psychology Research and Behavior Management, 14*, 1157–1170.

Ferguson, A.A., Khan, A.I., Abuzainah, B., Chaudhuri, D., et al. (2023). Clinical effectiveness of N-methyl-D-aspartate (NMDA) receptor antagonists in adult obsessive-compulsive disorder (OCD) treatment: A systematic review. *Cureus, 15*(4), e37833. doi:10.7759/cureus.c328

Fernández de la Cruz, L., Kolvenbach, S., Vidal-Ribas, P., Jassi, A., et al. (2016). Illness perception, help-seeking attitudes, and knowledge related to obsessive–compulsive disorder across different ethnic groups: A community survey. *Social Psychiatry and Psychiatric Epidemiology, 51*(3), 455–464.

Fineman, M.A. (1992). The Neutered Mother. *University of Miami Law Review, 46*, 653.

Five X More (2024). *The Black Maternity Experiences Survey*. www.nhsbmenetwork.org.uk/wp-content/uploads/2022/05/TheBlackMaternityExperienceReport.pdf

Flamarique, I., Plana, M.T., Castro-Fornieles, J., Borràs, R., Moreno, E., & Lázaro, L. (2019). Comparison of perfectionism dimensions in adolescents with anorexia nervosa or obsessive-compulsive disorder. *Journal of the Canadian Academy of Child and Adolescent Psychiatry, 28*(2), 45–54.

Forbes, N., Yang, L.C., & Lim, S. (2023). Intersectional discrimination and its impact on Asian American women's mental health: A mixed-methods scoping review. *Frontiers in Public Health, 11*, 993396. doi:10.3389/fpubh.2023.993396

Fornaro, M., Gabrielli, F., Albano, C., Fornaro, S., et al. (2009). Obsessive-compulsive disorder and related disorders: A comprehensive survey. *Annals of General Psychiatry, 8*, 13.

Freud S. (1909). Notes upon a case of obsessional neurosis. *Standard Edition 10*.

Gagliardi, M. (2021). How our caregivers shape who we are: The seven dimensions of attachment at the core of personality. *Frontiers in Psychology, 12*, 657628. doi:10.3389/fpsyg.2021.657628

Grados, M.A., Specht, M.W., Sung, H.M., & Fortune, D. (2013). Glutamate drugs and pharmacogenetics of OCD: A pathway-based exploratory approach. *Expert Opinion on Drug Discovery, 8*(12), 1515–1527.

Green, S.A., & Graham, B.M. (2022). Symptom fluctuation over the menstrual cycle in anxiety disorders, PTSD, and OCD: A systematic review. *Archives of Women's Mental Health, 25*, 71–85.

Greenberg, D., & Shefler, G. (2008). Ultra-orthodox rabbinic responses to religious obsessive-compulsive disorder. *The Israel Journal of Psychiatry and Related Sciences, 45*(3), 183–192.

Greenfield, M., & Darwin, Z. (2021). Trans and non-binary pregnancy, traumatic birth, and perinatal mental health: A scoping review. *International Journal of Transgender Health, 22*(1–2), 203–216.

Grekin, R., O'Hara, M.W., & Brock, R.L. (2021). A model of risk for perinatal post-traumatic stress symptoms. *Archives of Women's Mental Health, 24*, 259–270.

Griffiths, J., Lever Taylor, B., Morant, N., Bick, D., et al. (2019). A qualitative comparison of experiences of specialist mother and baby units versus general psychiatric wards. *BMC Psychiatry*, *19*(1), 401.

Grisham, J.R., Anderson, T.M., & Sachdev, P.S. (2008). Genetic and environmental influences on obsessive-compulsive disorder. *European Archives of Psychiatry and Clinical Neuroscience*, *258*, 107–116.

Guala, A., Folgori, G., Silvestri, M., Barbaglia, M., & Danesino, C. (2022). Vitamin B6 neonatal toxicity. *Case Reports in Pediatrics*, *2022*, 317135. doi:10.1155/2022/3171351I

Hale, T.W. (2021). *Hale's Medications & Mothers' Milk 2021: A Manual of Lactational Pharmacology* (19th edn). Springer.

Hewitt, P.L., & Flett, G.L. (1991). Perfectionism in the self and social contexts: Conceptualization, assessment, and association with psychopathology. *Journal of Personality and Social Psychology*, *60*(3), 456–470.

Hill, L., Rao, A., Artiga, S., & Ranji, U. (2024). Racial disparities in maternal and infant health: Current status and efforts to address them. www.kff.org/racial-equity-and-health-policy/issue-brief/racial-disparities-in-maternal-and-infant-health-current-status-and-efforts-to-address-them

HM Government (2021). *The Best Start in Life: A Vision for the 1,001 Critical Days*. The Leadsom Report. www.gov.uk/government/publications/the-best-start-for-life-a-vision-for-the-1001-critical-days

Hoang, T.H., Hsieh, W.J., Lee, B.A., Lukacena, K.M., & Tabb, K.M. (2022). Navigating pregnancy and the healthcare system during COVID-19: A qualitative study with perinatal women of color. *International Journal of Environmental Research and Public Health*, *19*(20), 13698. doi:10.3390/ijerph192013698

Hoang, T.H., Lee, B.A., Hsieh, W.J., Lukacena, K.M., & Tabb, K.M. (2023). Experiences of racial trauma among perinatal women of color in seeking healthcare services. *General Hospital Psychiatry*, *84*, 60–66.

House, S.J., Tripathi, S.P., Knight, B.T., Morris, N., Newport, D.J., & Stowe, Z.N. (2016). Obsessive-compulsive disorder in pregnancy and the postpartum period: Course of illness and obstetrical outcome. *Archives of Women's Mental Health*, *19*(1), 3–10.

International Obsessive Compulsive Disorder Foundation Genetics Collaborative and OCD Collaborative Genetics Association Studies (2018). Revealing the complex genetic architecture of obsessive-compulsive disorder using meta-analysis. *Molecular Psychiatry*, *23*(5), 1181–1188.

Jayarajah C.G. (2025). 'False positive': understanding pseudocyesis through old and new perspectives. *British Journal of Psychiatry*, 1–5 [Advance online publication]. doi:10.1192/bjp.2025.57

Jayarajah, C.G., & Seneviratne, T. (2016). Development of a mother and baby unit contraception assessment tool. *Archives of Women's Mental Health*, *19*(6), 1129–1140.

Joint Formulary Committee (2024). *British National Formulary 87*. BMJ Publishing and the Royal Pharmaceutical Society.

Karpinski, M., Mattina, G.F., & Steiner, M. (2017). Effect of gonadal hormones on neurotransmitters implicated in the pathophysiology of obsessive-compulsive disorder: A critical review. *Neuroendocrinology*, *105*(1), 1–16.

Kawamoto, T., & Furutani, K. (2018). The mediating role of intolerance of uncertainty on the relationships between perfectionism dimensions and psychological adjustment/maladjustment among mothers. *Personality and Individual Differences*, *122*, 62–67.

Kaye, W.H., Bulik, C.M., Thornton, L., Barbarich, N., & Masters, K. (2004). Comorbidity of anxiety disorders with anorexia and bulimia nervosa. *American Journal of Psychiatry*, *161*, 2215–2221.

Kerppola, J., Halme, N., Perälä, M.L., & Maija-Pietilä, A. (2019). Parental empowerment: Lesbian, gay, bisexual, trans or queer parents' perceptions of maternity and child healthcare. *International Journal of Nursing Practice*, *25*(5), e12755. doi:10.1111/ijn.12755

Kim, S., & Lee, S.H. (2020). Son preference and fertility decisions: Evidence from spatiotemporal variation in Korea. *Demography*, *57*(3), 927–951.

Kimmel, M. (2021). Care of the Homicidal Patient in Pregnancy or During the Postpartum Period: Managing Intrusive Thoughts; Special Considerations for OCD. In E. Cox (Ed.) *Women's Mood Disorders* (pp.273–281). Springer.

Korosi, A., & Baram, T.Z. (2009). The pathways from mother's love to baby's future. *Frontiers in Behavioral Neuroscience*, *3*, 27. doi:10.3389/neuro.08.027.2009

Koven, N.S., & Abry, A.W. (2015). The clinical basis of orthorexia nervosa: Emerging perspectives. *Neuropsychiatric Disease and Treatment*, *11*, 385–394.

Krebs, G., Waszczuk, M.A., Zavos, H.M., Bolton, D., & Eley, T.C. (2015). Genetic and environmental influences on obsessive-compulsive behaviour across development: A longitudinal twin study. *Psychological Medicine*, *45*(7), 1539–1549.

Kuty-Pachecka, M. (2021). Sexual obsessions in obsessive-compulsive disorder: Definitions, models and cognitive-behavioural therapy. *Psychiatria Polska*, *55*(1), 39–52.

Lapidus, K.A., Kopell, B.H., Ben-Haim, S., Rezai, A.R., & Goodman, W.K. (2013). History of psychosurgery: A psychiatrist's perspective. *World Neurosurgery*, *80*(3–4), S27.e116. doi:10.1016/j.wneu.2013.02.053

Laughter, M.R., Anderson, J.B., Maymone, M.B.C., & Kroumpouzos, G. (2023). Psychology of aesthetics: Beauty, social media, and body dysmorphic disorder. *Clinical Dermatology*, *41*(1), 28–32.

Lee, M.A., Schoppe-Sullivan, S.J., & Kamp Dush, C.M. (2012). Parenting perfectionism and parental adjustment. *Personality and Individual Difference*, *52*(3), 454–457.

Liu, M., Kim, D.W., Zeng, H., & Anderson, D.J. (2022). Make war not love: The neural substrate underlying a state-dependent switch in female social behavior. *Neuron*, *110*(5), 841–856.

Lochner, C., & Stein, D. (2011). Gender in obsessive-compulsive disorder and obsessive-compulsive spectrum disorders. *Archives of Women's Mental Health* *4*, 19–26.

Lochner, C., McGregor, N., Hemmings, S., Harvey, B.H., et al. (2016). Symmetry symptoms in obsessive-compulsive disorder: Clinical and genetic correlates. *Brazilian Journal of Psychiatry*, *38*(1), 17–23.

Lorberbaum, J.P., Newman, J.D., Dubno, J.R., Horwitz, A.R., et al. (1999). Feasibility of using fMRI to study mothers responding to infant cries. *Depression and Anxiety*, *10*(3), 99–104.

Mackle, T., Colodro-Conde, L., de Dassel, T., Braun, A., et al. (2023). 'Echoes of a dark past' is a history of maternal childhood maltreatment a perinatal risk factor for pregnancy and postpartum trauma experiences? A longitudinal study. *BMC Pregnancy and Childbirth*, *23*(1), 397. doi:10.1186/s12884-023-05714-2

Mahaffey, B.L., Levinson, A., Preis, H., & Lobel, M. (2022). Elevated risk for obsessive–compulsive symptoms in women pregnant during the COVID-19 pandemic. *Archives of Women's Mental Health*, *25*, 367–376.

Mahjani, B., Bey, K., Boberg, J., & Burton, C. (2021). Genetics of obsessive-compulsive disorder. *Psychological Medicine*, *51*(13), 2247–2259.

Maiti, R., Mishra, A., Srinivasan, A., & Mishra, B.R. (2023). Pharmacological augmentation of serotonin reuptake inhibitors in patients with obsessive-compulsive disorder: A network meta-analysis. *Acta Psychiatrica Scandinavica*, *148*(1), 19–31.

Mak, L., Streiner, D.L., & Steiner, M. (2015). Is serotonin transporter polymorphism (5-HTTLPR) allele status a predictor for obsessive-compulsive disorder? A meta-analysis. *Archives of Women's Mental Health*, *18*(3) 435–445.

Mamun, A., Biswas, T., Scott, J., Sly, P.D., et al. (2023). Adverse childhood experiences, the risk of pregnancy complications and adverse pregnancy outcomes: A systematic review and meta-analysis. *BMJ Open*, *13*(8), e063826. doi:10.1136/bmjopen-2022-063826

Marazziti, D., Falaschi, V., Lombardi, A., Mungai, F., & Dell'Osso, L. (2015). Stalking: A neurobiological perspective. *Rivista di Psichiatria*, *50*(1), 12–18.

Martínez-García, M., Paternina-Die, M., Desco, M., Vilarroya, O., & Carmona, S. (2021). Characterizing the brain structural adaptations across the motherhood transition. *Frontiers in Global Women's Health*, *2*, 742775. doi:10.3389/fgwh.2021.742775

Mataix-Cols, D., & van den Heuvel, O.A. (2012). Neuroanatomy of Obsessive Compulsive and Related Disorders. In G. Steketee (Ed.) *The Oxford Handbook of Obsessive Compulsive and Spectrum Disorders* (pp.127–144). Oxford Academic.

Mataix-Cols, D., Boman, M., Monzani, B., Rück, C., et al. (2013). Population-based, multigenerational family clustering study of obsessive-compulsive disorder. *JAMA Psychiatry*, *70*(7), 709–717.

Mathes, B.M., Morabito, D.M., & Schmidt, N.B. (2019). Epidemiological and clinical gender differences in OCD. *Current Psychiatry Reports*, *21*(5), 36. doi:10.1007/s11920-019-1015-2

Mattheisen, M., Samuels, J.F., Wang, Y., Greenberg, B.D., et al. (2015). Genome-wide association study in obsessive-compulsive disorder: Results from the OCGAS. *Molecular Psychiatry*, *20*(3), 337–344.

Mattina, G.F., & Steiner, M. (2016). The need for inclusion of sex and age of onset variables in genetic association studies of obsessive-compulsive disorder: Overview. *Progress in Neuro-psychopharmacology & Biological Psychiatry*, *67*, 107–116.

MBRRACE-UK (2025). *Saving Lives, Improving Mothers' Care: Lessons Learned to Inform Maternity Care from the UK and Ireland Confidential Enquiries into Maternal Deaths and Morbidity 2021–23*. MBRRACE-UK. www.npeu.ox.ac.uk/mbrrace-uk/reports/maternal-reports

McManus, M.A., Hargreaves, P., Rainbow, L., & Alison, L.J. (2013). Paraphilias: Definition, diagnosis and treatment. *F1000Prime Reports*, *5*, 36. doi:10.12703/P5-36

Mind (2023). Symptoms of OCD. https://www.mind.org.uk/information-support/types-of-mental-health-problems/obsessive-compulsive-disorder-ocd/symptoms-of-ocd

Modleski, T. (2015). *The Woman Who Knew Too Much: Hitchcock and Feminist Theory* (3rd edn). Routledge.

Moritz, S., Kempke, S., Luyten, P., Randjbar, S., & Jelinek, L. (2011). Was Freud partly right on obsessive-compulsive disorder (OCD)? Investigation of latent aggression in OCD. *Psychiatry Research*, *187*(1–2), 180–184.

Mowrer, O.H., & Lamoreaux, R.R. (1946). Fear as an intervening variable in avoidance conditioning. *Journal of Comparative Psychology*, *39*(1), 29–50.

Nakao, T., Okada, K., & Kanba, S. (2014). Neurobiological model of obsessive-compulsive disorder: Evidence from recent neuropsychological and neuro-imaging findings. *Psychiatry and Clinical Neurosciences*, *68*(8), 587–605.

Nasiri, K., Czuzoj-Shulman, N., & Abenhaim, H.A. (2021). Association between obsessive-compulsive disorder and obstetrical and neonatal outcomes in the USA: A population-based cohort study. *Archives of Women's Mental Health*, *24*, 971–978.

National Autistic Society (n.d.). Obsessive compulsive disorder (OCD). https://www.autism.org.uk/advice-and-guidance/mental-health/ocd

National Institutes of Health (1994). *Outreach Notebook for the NIH Guidelines on the Inclusion of Women and Minorities as Subjects in Clinical Research*. National Institutes of Health.

Nedeljkovic, M., Moulding, R., Foroughi, E., Kyrios, M., & Doron, G. (2012). Cultural Issues in Understanding and Treating Obsessive Compulsive and Spectrum Disorders. In G. Steketee (Ed.) *The Oxford Handbook of Obsessive Compulsive and Spectrum Disorders* (pp.497–518). Oxford University Press.

Nezgovorova, V., Reid, J., Fineberg, N.A., & Hollander, E. (2022). Optimizing first line treatments for adults with OCD. *Comprehensive Psychiatry*, *115*, 152305. doi:10.1016/j.comppsych.2022.152305

NHS (2024). Infections in pregnancy that may affect your baby. www.nhs.uk/pregnancy/keeping-well/infections-that-may-affect-your-baby

NHS England (2016). *Implementing the Five Year Forward View for Mental Health*. www.england.nhs.uk/wp-content/uploads/2016/07/fyfv-mh.pdf

NHS England (n.d.). Maternal mental health services. www.england.nhs.uk/mental-health/perinatal/maternal-mental-health-services

NHS Mental Health Taskforce (2016). *Five Year Forward View for Mental Health*. www.england.nhs.uk/wp-content/uploads/2016/02/Mental-Health-Taskforce-FYFV-final.pdf

NICE (2005). Obsessive-compulsive disorder and body dysmorphic disorder: Treatment. Clinical guideline (CG31). www.nice.org.uk/Guidance/CG31

NICE (2014). Antenatal and postnatal mental health: Clinical management and service guidance. Clinical guideline (CG192). www.nice.org.uk/guidance/cg192

NICE (2021). Deep brain stimulation for chronic, severe, treatment resistant obsessive compulsive disorder in adults. Interventional procedure guidance (IPG693). www.nice.org.uk/guidance/ipg693

Nicolini, H., Salin-Pascual, R., Cabrera, B., & Lanzagorta, N. (2017). Influence of culture in obsessive-compulsive disorder and its treatment. *Current Psychiatry Reviews*, *13*(4), 285–292.

Nooyi, I. (2021). *My Life in Full: Work, Family, and Our Future*. Piatkus.

Oakley, A. (1974). *Woman's Work: The Housewife, Past and Present*. Pantheon.

Oberbeck, A., Stengler, K., & Steinberg, H. (2013). Die Geschichte der Zwangserkrankung: Ihre Stellung im Wandel der psychiatrischen Formenlehre bis Anfang des 20. Jahrhunderts [On the history of obsessive-compulsive disorders: Their place in the nosological classifications up to the beginning of the 20th century]. *Fortschritte der Neurologie-Psychiatrie*, *81*(12), 706–714.

OCD-UK (2025a). Hoarding disorder. www.OCDuk.org/related-disorders/hoarding-disorder

OCD-UK (2025b). What are obsessions? www.OCDuk.org/OCD/obsessions

OCD-UK (2025c). The history of OCD. www.OCDuk.org/OCD/history-of-OCD

O'Hara, L., Smith, E.R., Barlow, J., Livingstone, N., et al. (2019). Video feedback for parental sensitivity and attachment security in children under five years. *Cochrane Database of Systematic Reviews, 11*(11), CD012348. doi:10.1002/14651858.CD012348.pub2

Orbach, S., & Rubin, H. (2014). *Two for the Price of One: The Impact of Body Image during Pregnancy and after Birth*. Government Equalities Office. www.gov.uk/government/publications/two-for-the-price-of-one

Ortiz, G.G.R., Tapia, C.J.R., Martínez, B.A.E., & Icaza, D. (2022). Mediating mechanisms of perfectionism: Clinical comorbidity of OCD and ED. *Frontiers in Psychiatry, 13*, 908926. doi:10.3389/fpsyt.2022.908926

Pederson, D.R., Bailey, H.N., Tarabulsy, G.M., Bento, S., & Moran, G. (2014). Understanding sensitivity: Lessons learned from the legacy of Mary Ainsworth. *Attachment and Human Development, 16*(3), 261–270.

Pedrucci, G. (2020). The entanglement of mothers and religions: An introduction. *Open Theology, 6*(1), 202–205.

Pellegrini, L., Fineberg, N.A., O'Connor, S., De Souza, A.M.F.L.P., et al. (2025). Single-dose (10 mg) psilocybin reduces symptoms in adults with obsessive-compulsive disorder: A pharmacological challenge study. *Comprehensive Psychiatry, 142*, 152619. doi:10.1016/j.comppsych.2025.152619

Phillips, K.A., & Kelly, M.M. (2021). Body dysmorphic disorder: Clinical overview and relationship to obsessive-compulsive disorder. *Focus (American Psychiatric Publishing), 19*(4), 413–419.

Pinciotti, C.M., Nuñez, M., Riemann, B.C., & Bailey, B.E. (2022). Clinical presentation and treatment trajectory of gender minority patients with obsessive-compulsive disorder. *Journal of Cognitive Psychotherapy, 36*(1), 42–59.

Pontillo, M., Zanna, V., Demaria, F., Averna, R., et al. (2022). Orthorexia nervosa, eating disorders, and obsessive-compulsive disorder: A selective review of the last seven years. *Journal of Clinical Medicine, 11*(20), 6134. doi:10.3390/jcm11206134

Postorino, V., Kerns, C.M., Vivanti, G., Bradshaw, J., Siracusano, M., & Mazzone, L. (2017). Anxiety disorders and obsessive-compulsive disorder in individuals with autism spectrum disorder. *Current Psychiatry Reports, 19*(12), 92.

Pryzgoda, J., & Chrisler, J.C. (2000). Definitions of gender and sex: The subtleties of meaning. *Sex Roles, 43*, 553–569.

Purty, A., Nestadt, G., Samuels, J.F., & Viswanath, B. (2019). Genetics of obsessive-compulsive disorder. *Indian Journal of Psychiatry, 61*(Suppl 1), S37–S42.

Rapinesi, C., Kotzalidis, G.D., Ferracuti, S., Sani, G., Girardi, P., & Del Casale, A. (2019). Brain stimulation in obsessive-compulsive disorder (OCD): A systematic review. *Current Neuropharmacology, 17*(8), 787–807.

Ravi, M., Stevens, J.S., & Michopoulos, V. (2019). Neuroendocrine pathways underlying risk and resilience to PTSD in women. *Frontiers in Neuroendocrinology, 55*, 100790. doi:10.1016/j.yfrne.2019.100790

Reid, J.E., Laws, K.R., Drummond, L., Vismara, M., et al. (2021). Cognitive behavioural therapy with exposure and response prevention in the treatment of obsessive-compulsive disorder: A systematic review and meta-analysis of randomised controlled trials. *Comprehensive Psychiatry*, *106*, 152223. doi:10.1016/j.comppsych.2021.152223

Rossell, S.L., Labuschagne, I., Castle, D.J., & Toh, W.L. (2020). Delusional themes in body dysmorphic disorder (BDD): Comparisons with psychotic disorders and non-clinical controls. *Psychiatry Research*, *284*, 112694. doi:10.1016/j.psychres.2019.112694

Royal College of Obstetricians and Gynaecologists (n.d.). *Policy Position: Racial and Ethnic Equality in Women's Health*. www.rcog.org.uk/about-us/campaigning-and-opinions/position-statements/policy-position-racial-and-ethnic-equality-in-women-s-health

Royal College of Psychiatrists (2020). *Assessment and Management of Adults and Children in Cases of Fabricated or Induced Illness (FII)*. www.rcpsych.ac.uk/docs/default-source/improving-care/better-mh-policy/college-reports/cr223.pdf

Royal College of Psychiatrists (2021). *Perinatal Mental Health Services: Recommendations for the Provision of Services for Childbearing Women*. www.rcpsych.ac.uk/docs/default-source/improving-care/better-mh-policy/college-reports/college-report-cr232---perinatal-mental-heath-services.pdf

Royal College of Psychiatrists (2023a). *Infant and Early Childhood Mental Health: The Case for Action*. www.rcpsych.ac.uk/improving-care/campaigning-for-better-mental-health-policy/college-reports/2023-college-reports/infant-and-early-childhood-mental-health--the-case-for-action-(cr238)

Royal College of Psychiatrists (2023b). *Stalking*. Psychiatrists Support Service information guide. www.rcpsych.ac.uk/docs/default-source/members/supporting-you/pss/pss-guide-11-stalking.pdf

Royal College of Psychiatrists (2025). *Co-occurring Substance Use and Mental Health Disorders (CoSUM)*. College Report CR243. www.rcpsych.ac.uk/docs/default-source/improving-care/better-mh-policy/college-reports/college-report-cr243---cosum.pdf

Royal Foundation (n.d.). Early childhood. https://royalfoundation.com/early-childhood

Samuels, J.F. (2009). Recent advances in the genetics of obsessive-compulsive disorder. *Current Psychiatry Reports*, *11*(4), 277–282.

Sayers, J. (1993). *Mothers of Psychoanalysis: Helene Deutsch, Karen Horney, Anna Freud, Melanie Klein* (Abridged edn). W.W. Norton & Co.

Schafer, R. (1974). Problems in Freud's psychology of women. *Journal of the American Psychoanalytic Association*, *22*(3), 459–485.

Schoppe-Sullivan, S.J., Yavorsky, J.E., Bartholomew, M.K., Sullivan, J.M., et al. (2017). Doing gender online: New mothers' psychological characteristics, Facebook use, and depressive symptoms. *Sex Roles*, *76*(5), 276–289.

Seeman, M.V. (2014). Pseudocyesis, delusional pregnancy, and psychosis: The birth of a delusion. *World Journal of Clinical Cases*, *2*(8), 338–344.

Shannon, Lyttanya (2021). 'The Black Maternity Scandal.' *Dispatches*. Channel 4, 29 March 2021.

Sharma, A., & Shrivastava, D. (2022). Psychological problems related to infertility. *Cureus*, *14*(10), e30320. doi:10.7759/cureus.30320

Sharma, V. (2018). Pharmacotherapy of postpartum obsessive-compulsive disorder: A systematic review. *Expert Review of Neurotherapeutics*, *18*(12), 925–931.

Shih, H.C., Kuo, M.E., Wu, C.W., Chao, Y.P., Huang, H.W., & Huang, C.M. (2022). The neurobiological basis of love: A meta-analysis of human functional neuroimaging studies of maternal and passionate love. *Brain Sciences*, *12*(7), 830. doi:10.3390/brainsci12070830

Sicard, A., Redersdorff, S., Darnon, C., & Martinot, D. (2021). Dealing with a crisis: Does Covid-19 promote traditional gender roles? *Psycholica Belgica*, *61*(1), 212–223.

Signori, J.P.S., do Canto, G.C., Roza, T.H., de Borba Telles, L.E., & de Almeida Fleck, M.P. (2022). Stalking in clinical psychiatry: When the doctor becomes the victim. *Brazilian Journal of Psychiatry*, *44*(4), 464–465.

Sinopoli, V.M., Burton, C.L., Kronenberg, S., & Arnold, P.D. (2017). A review of the role of serotonin system genes in obsessive-compulsive disorder. *Neuroscience and Biobehavioral Reviews*, *80*, 372–381.

Slepneva, N., Basich-Pease, G., Reid, L., Frank, A.C., et al. (2024). Therapeutic DBS for OCD suppresses the default mode network. *Human Brain Mapping*, *45*(18), e70106. doi:10.1002/hbm.70106

Smith, M.M., Sherry, S.B., Mushquash, A.R., Saklofske, D.H., Gautreau, C., & Nealis, L.J. (2017). Perfectionism erodes social self-esteem and generates depressive symptoms: Studying mother–daughter dyads using a daily diary design with longitudinal follow-up. *Journal of Research in Personality*, *71*, 72–79.

Spurlock, E.J., & Pickler, R.H. (2024). Birth experience among black women in the United States: A qualitative meta-synthesis. *Journal of Midwifery & Women's Health*, *69*(5), 697–717.

Srinivasan, A. (2021). *The Right to Sex*. Bloomsbury.

Stahl, S.M. (2020). *Prescriber's Guide: Stahl's Essential Psychopharmacology* (7th edn). Cambridge University Press.

Starcevic, V., Eslick, G.D., Viswasam, K., & Berle, D. (2020). Symptoms of obsessive-compulsive disorder during pregnancy and the postpartum period: A systematic review and meta-analysis. *Psychiatric Quarterly*, *91*, 965–981.

Stengel, C., Sanches, C., Toba, M.N., & Valero-Cabré, A. (2022). Things you wanted to know (but might have been afraid to ask) about how and why to explore and modulate brain plasticity with non-invasive neurostimulation technologies. *Revue Neurologique*, *178*(8), 826–844.

Stephenson, L.A., Macdonald, A.J.D., Seneviratne, G., Waites, F., & Pawlby, S. (2018). Mother and baby units matter: Improved outcomes for both. *BJPsych Open*, *4*(3), 119–125. doi:10.1192/bjo.2018.7

Stevens, N.R., Heath, N.M., Lillis, T.A., McMinn, K., Tirone, V., & Sha'ini, M. (2018). Examining the effectiveness of a coordinated perinatal mental health care model using an intersectional-feminist perspective. *Journal of Behavioral Medicine*, *41*, 627–640.

Stewart, S.E., Yu, D., Scharf, J.M., Neale, B.M., et al. (2013). Genome-wide association study of obsessive-compulsive disorder. *Molecular Psychiatry*, *18*(7), 788–798.

Tasca, C., Rapetti, M., Carta, M.G., & Fadda, B. (2012). Women and hysteria in the history of mental health. *Clinical Practice and Epidemiology in Mental Health*, *8*, 110–119. doi:10.2174/1745017901208010110

Taylor, D.M., Barnes, T.R.E., & Young, A.H. (2018). *The Maudsley Prescribing Guidelines in Psychiatry* (13th edn). John Wiley & Sons.

Thamby, A., & Jaisoorya, T.S. (2019). Antipsychotic augmentation in the treatment of obsessive-compulsive disorder. *Indian Journal of Psychiatry*, *61*(Suppl 1), S51–S57. doi:10.4103/psychiatry.IndianJPsychiatry_519_18

Tolin, D.F., & Worden, B.L. (2012). Combining Pharmacotherapy and Psychological Treatments for OCD. In G. Steketee (Ed.) *The Oxford Handbook of Obsessive Compulsive and Spectrum Disorders* (pp.365–376). Oxford Academic.

Tone, A., & Koziol, M. (2018). (F)ailing women in psychiatry: Lessons from a painful past. *Canadian Medical Association Journal*, *190*(20), E624–E625.

Tosato, S., Albert, U., Tomassi, S., Iasevoli, F., et al. (2017). A systematized review of atypical antipsychotics in pregnant women: Balancing between risks of untreated illness and risks of drug-related adverse effects. *Journal of Clinical Psychiatry*, *78*(5), e477–e489.

Tran, N., Callaway, L., Shen, S., Biswas, T., et al. (2022). Screening for adverse childhood experiences in antenatal care settings: A scoping review. *Australian & New Zealand Journal of Obstetrics & Gynaecology*, *62*(5), 626–634.

Trede, K., Baldessarini, R.J., Viguera, A.C., & Bottero, A. (2009). Treatise on insanity in pregnant, postpartum, and lactating women (1858) by Louis-Victor Marcé: A commentary. *Harvard Review of Psychiatry*, *17*(2), 157–165.

Tyagi, H., Apergis-Schoute, A.M., Akram, H., Foltynie, T., et al. (2019). A randomized trial directly comparing ventral capsule and anteromedial subthalamic nucleus stimulation in obsessive-compulsive disorder: Clinical and imaging evidence for dissociable effects. *Biological Psychiatry*, *85*(9), 726–734.

UNICEF UK (n.d.). The Baby Friendly Initiative. www.unicef.org.uk/babyfriendly

van Grootheest, D.S., Cath, D.C., Beekman, A.T., & Boomsma, D.I. (2005). Twin studies on obsessive-compulsive disorder: A review. *Twin Research and Human Genetics*, *8*(5), 450–458.

van Westen, M., Rietveld, E., Figee, M., & Denys, D. (2015). Clinical outcome and mechanisms of deep brain stimulation for obsessive-compulsive disorder. *Current Behavioral Neuroscience Reports*, *2*(2), 41–48.

Vella-Zarb, R.A., Cohen, J.N., McCabe, R.E., & Rowa, K. (2017). Differentiating sexual thoughts in obsessive-compulsive disorder from paraphilias and non-paraphilic sexual disorders. *Cognitive and Behavioral Practice*, *24*(3), 342–352.

Walker, R., Blackie, M., & Nedeljkovic, M. (2021). Fathers' experience of perinatal obsessive–compulsive symptoms: A systematic literature review. *Clinical Child and Family Psychology Review*, *24*(3), 529–541.

Weiss, M., Baerg, E., Wisebord, S., & Temple, J. (1995). The influence of gonadal hormones on periodicity of obsessive-compulsive disorder. *Canadian Journal of Psychiatry*, *40*, 4, 205–207.

Welldon, E.V. (1992). *Mother, Madonna, Whore: The Idealisation and Denigration of Motherhood*. Routledge.

Wilcox, A.J., Weinberg, C.R., & Baird, D.D. (1995). Timing of sexual intercourse in relation to ovulation: Effects on the probability of conception, survival of the pregnancy, and sex of the baby. *New England Journal of Medicine*, *333*(23), 1517–1521.

Williams, H. (2013, 19 December). Six facts about elephant families. *Independent*. www.independent.co.uk/voices/comment/six-facts-about-elephant-families-9015298.html

Williams, M., Powers, M., Yun, Y.G., & Foa, E. (2010). Minority participation in randomized controlled trials for obsessive-compulsive disorder. *Journal of Anxiety Disorders*, *24*(2), 171–177.

Winnicott, D.W. (1967). *Playing and Reality*. Routledge.

Women's Aid (2019). *Supporting Women and Babies after Domestic Abuse: A Toolkit for Domestic Abuse Specialists.* www.womensaid.org.uk/wp-content/uploads/2019/12/Supporting-women-and-babies-after-domestic-abuse.pdf

Yehuda, R., & Lehrner, A. (2018). Intergenerational transmission of trauma effects: Putative role of epigenetic mechanisms. *World Psychiatry*, *17*(3), 243–257.

Yilmaz, H., Karakuş, G., Tamam, L., Demirkol, M.E., Namlı, Z., & Yeşiloğlu, C. (2020). Association of orthorexic tendencies with obsessive-compulsive symptoms, eating attitudes and exercise. *Neuropsychiatric Diseases and Treatment*, *16*, 3035–3044.

Yuvaci, H.U., Yazici, E., Yazici, A.B., & Cevrioglu, S. (2019). How often do women use non-drug treatment methods for psychiatric symptoms during pregnancy and postpartum periods? *Mental Illness*, *11*(1), 7988. doi:10.4081/mi.2019.7988

Zagaria, A., Vacca, M., Cerolini, S., Ballesio, A., & Lombardo, C. (2022). Associations between orthorexia, disordered eating, and obsessive-compulsive symptoms: A systematic review and meta-analysis. *International Journal of Eating Disorders*, *55*(3), 295–312.

Zambaldi, C.F., Cantilino, A., Montenegro, A.C., Paes, J.A., de Albuquerque, T.L.C., & Sougey, E.B. (2009). Postpartum obsessive-compulsive disorder: Prevalence and clinical characteristics. *Comprehensive Psychiatry*, *50*(6), 503–509.

Zeki, S. (2007). The neurobiology of love. *FEBS Letters*, *581*(14), 2575–2579.

Subject Index

Author Index